ELDER ABUSE PREVENTION

Elder Abuse Prevention

Emerging Trends and Promising Strategies

LISA NERENBERG, MSW, MPH

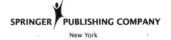
SPRINGER PUBLISHING COMPANY
New York

Springer Publishing Company, LLC
11 West 42nd Street
New York, NY 10036
www.springerpub.com

Acquisitions Editor: Sheri W. Sussman
Production Editor: Rosanne Lugtu
Cover design: Joanne E. Honigman
Composition: Publication Services, Inc.

07 08 09 10/5 4 3 2 1

Library of Congress Cataloging-in-Publication Data

Nerenberg, Lisa.
  Elder abuse prevention : emerging trends and promising strategies / Lisa Nerenberg.
    p. cm.
  ISBN 978-0-8261-0327-7 (hardcover : alk. paper)
  1. Older people--Abuse of--Prevention. 2. Abused elderly--Services for. I. Title.

HV6626.3.N47 2008
362.6--dc22
                        2007041128

Printed in the United States of America by Bang Printing.

This book is dedicated to my husband, Daniel Woodard,
and my sister, Lynne Nerenberg, for their unwavering support,
love, and insights. And in loving memory of my parents,
Toby and Rush Nerenberg, whose values continue to guide me.

Author Biography

Lisa Nerenberg, MSW, MPH is a consultant in elder abuse prevention. Previously, she directed the San Francisco Consortium for Elder Abuse Prevention at the Institute on Aging, which was one of the first elder abuse prevention programs in the country. Under her leadership, the Consortium piloted some of the country's first abuse prevention services and interventions, including a multidisciplinary team, a counseling program and support group for victims, and culturally specific outreach. She has provided training and technical assistance to local, state, and national organizations; developed comprehensive training curricula; delivered keynote addresses, moderated panels, and made presentations at hundreds of professional forums in the United States and Canada. Ms. Nerenberg has testified before Congressional committees and served on governmental advisory committees and panels. She has authored dozens of articles, chapters, and publications on such far-ranging topics as coalition building, the role of culture and gender in elder abuse, financial abuse and the special needs of financial crime victims, daily money management, and the role of the civil and criminal justice systems in elder abuse prevention. A special area of interest is cross-disciplinary exchange among professionals in the fields of aging, criminal justice, victim-witness assistance, health and mental health, domestic violence, and adult protective services. Her Web site (http://www.lisanerenberg.com/) and blog (http://preventelderabuse.blogspot.com) address cutting-edge issues in the field today.

Contents

Preface

If, as some suggest, the moral test of a society is how it treats its elders, the shocking accounts of elder abuse that are increasingly hitting the headlines cast us in very grim light. Almost daily, we hear about frail, abandoned elders languishing in filth; adult children plundering their parents' estates; and predators preying upon the sick, disabled, and lonesome.

But societies are also defined by how they respond to problems, and in the quarter-century since elder abuse first emerged into the public's consciousness, professionals, advocates, and concerned citizens have demonstrated remarkable ingenuity and determination. They have scoured the literature from far-ranging disciplines in search of explanations and strategies, forged alliances with unlikely partners, and grappled with such slippery questions as when to intervene in the lives of elders who do not want help.

This book describes what has been accomplished and what remains to be done to stop abuse, treat its effects, and ensure justice. It further addresses the broader need to fortify our long-term care, protective service, and legal systems to meet the new and imminent demands of a burgeoning elderly population. In short, it is about making our communities safer places to grow old.

In writing the book, I have drawn from the published literature, from observations shared by colleagues, and, to a great extent, from my own experiences over the last twenty-four years. For most of that time, I directed the San Francisco Consortium for Elder Abuse Prevention, one of the first programs to address elder abuse. During those years, and in the seven years since starting a private practice, I have worked with hundreds of agencies, state and local coalitions, planning councils, and multidisciplinary teams across the United States and Canada. No two are quite alike, yet neither are they very different.

San Francisco's response to elder abuse began in 1981, when the House Select Committee on Aging held one of its groundbreaking hearings here, and several local professionals were invited to testify. The event sparked interest and prompted the local Coalition of Agencies Serving the Elderly (CASE) to assign a task force to explore the issue further.

What happened next reads like a textbook case study in community organizing. The task force developed a questionnaire survey for local agencies, asking them about abuse victims they had served during the past year, their abusers, the circumstances, and what the agencies had done. Although the survey only generated 146 cases, it was the largest study of its kind at the time and yielded valuable insight into victims' service needs. More importantly, it pointed out that no single agency was equipped to meet all those needs, which ranged from medical treatment to legal assistance. The task force called for agencies to work together and designed a model, which became the blueprint for the San Francisco Consortium for Elder Abuse Prevention. Key features were a steering committee, a coordinating agency, advocacy and training committees, and a multidisciplinary case review team. They charged Mount Zion Hospital with coordinating the new program.

That was in 1983. I had just moved to San Francisco from Minnesota, where I had recently finished my graduate coursework in public health and social work. I was looking for an unpaid internship, and someone referred me to Mount Zion. Because the hospital had not received any funding to launch the new elder abuse program, I was a perfect candidate for the job. Susan Garbuio, one of the driving forces behind the task force and an innovator in aging services, "hired" me.

One of my first responsibilities was to organize and provide staff support to the Consortium's multidisciplinary team, which met monthly to review complex cases. Because I had never worked with elders and had not had any courses on aging in grad school, it was not long before I was in over my head. Team members rattled off terms like IADLs, MSSP, MMSE, 5150s, APS, TIAs, and ADHCs; and a police officer grilled a social worker about whether a perpetrator had struck her client with an open hand or closed fist. When someone reported that a client knew who the last president was but could not count backward by sevens, I felt sure I had stumbled through the looking glass.

I appealed to Susan for help. She explained what she could and directed me to others on the team to fill in the blanks. After many calls, I came to the realization that there was no single point during any meeting when everyone around the table understood what was going on. From then on, I took it upon myself to interrupt and ask for explanations. In doing so, I discovered that embedded in all those cryptic codes and riddles were the secrets to helping victims. I started picking up the jargon and learned that the difference between striking someone with a flat hand and closed fist might determine whether criminal charges applied and whether the victim's cooperation was needed to move forward. The inability to count backward or remember presidents suggested impairments that heightened vulnerability and dictated what interventions were needed. When I noticed others around the table staring at me, I knew it was my cue to interrupt on their behalf.

There is nothing quite as contagious as the creative energy that flows when service providers swap ideas and information to help clients. But our discussions were not limited to clients; team members voiced their frustrations, identified unmet needs, and prodded each other to tackle new problems and cases. We shared successes, commiserated on failures, and railed in outrage when systems failed. Team members tried out new approaches. Our local legal assistance to the elderly program became one of the first in the country to use domestic violence restraining orders to protect elderly victims from abusive offspring as well as partners. Staff of a daily money management program explained how clients were cheated and scammed and instructed us in how to reduce their risk. Getting to know police, nurses, lawyers, doctors, mental health professionals, and prosecutors was personally and professionally enriching, and these early experiences instilled in me a fascination with interdisciplinary exchange and program development.

Not long after the Consortium was up and running, we started getting requests from other communities and coalitions for help, and, in 1985, received the first of several grants from the Administration on Aging, Department of Health and Human Services, to provide training, consultation, and technical assistance. Some of the programs I worked with, like our Consortium, were inspired by government initiatives, whereas others were mandated, launched in response to local tragedies, or started because someone got a grant. Regardless of their origins, the programs were remarkably similar in several respects. All recognized that preventing elder abuse required a multidisciplinary response. The agencies and disciplines represented at the table were essentially the same regardless of whether the table was in Illinois or New York. So too were the challenges they faced, the jargon members used, and the services their clients needed.

Multidisciplinary exchange and cooperation are not always easy. Professional outlooks and opinions reflect deeply rooted commitments, values, and ideologies. When professionals from diverse backgrounds disagree on how to handle cases or address systemic problems, sparks may fly or fingers point. But these exchanges are a necessary part of ensuring that clients benefit from the full range of available options. The goal of multidisciplinary exchange is not to reach consensus but rather to ensure that all points of view are considered and to provide a system of checks and balances. Eventually, as service providers come to understand the restrictions and limitations their colleagues operate under, these exchanges become more collegial.

As the field developed, we drew from an increasingly wide array of disciplines and service delivery models. The perspectives, strategies, and resources that other disciplines contribute have enriched our field, but growth has not come without conflict. Ideological differences and competition for scarce resources have led to turfism and "clashing paradigms." "New and improved" models have been advanced and credited with trumping those that came before.

But elder abuse defies one-size-fits-all solutions. I believe that the best way to overcome competition and conflict is to help diverse groups understand one another. That is the goal of this book. It is intended to help readers better understand and appreciate the rich, if sometimes discordant, patchwork of theory and practice that defines our field. It is for those who work in the fields of aging, Adult Protective Services (APS), dementia care, mental health, legal aid, victim-witness assistance, domestic violence, law enforcement, and others. It is for both newcomers to the field and veterans. It is intended to augment these workers' repertoires of skills and lead to greater interdisciplinary collaboration and coordination. It is also for advocates, program developers, and concerned citizens, who want to improve their agencies,' communities,' tribes,' or states' responses to the problem.

For many years, the San Francisco Consortium had a committee called WE ARE FAMILY, which focused on the special needs of African American elders. The group had a tradition that I found very moving. Outreach events began with a *libation*, a prayer used in traditional African life to keep families linked to their legacies and honor those who came before. Members of the audience were invited to shout out the names of their ancestors, elders, and mentors. Following in that tradition, I would like to invoke the names of a few individuals who influenced and inspired me. Rosalie Wolf, a friend and mentor, embodied the spirit of collaboration and inclusiveness. She also believed that research, practice, and policy must be intertwined, and, to that end, she conducted numerous practice-focused studies and founded the *Journal of Elder Abuse & Neglect*, the National Committee for the Prevention of Elder Abuse, and the International Network for the Prevention of Elder Abuse. Jack McKay, also a friend and mentor, was a founding member of the San Francisco Consortium and a pioneer in the field of aging and daily money management. A strong believer in collaborative planning, he urged us to envision the future, even during times of retrenchment, when the possibility of growth or change seemed remote. "Know what you want," he would often say, "and you'll be surprised by what you can achieve."

Acknowledgments

I am indebted to the many friends and colleagues who have made my work both professionally and personally enriching. Special thanks to Mary Joy Quinn, who encouraged and inspired me to write this book, and to Eileen Goldman, for her careful read, insights, and feedback. I would also like to thank the many others who shared their ideas, case examples, and knowledge, including Melissa Anderson, Mary Counihan, Debbie Deem, Arlene Groh, Casey Gwinn, Judy Hitchcock, Diana Koin, Shawna Reeves Nourzaie, Nancy Rasch, Mary Twomey, members of the San Francisco Consortium, and colleagues around the world.

CHAPTER ONE

Eight Trends Shaping Practice

INTRODUCTION

As is the case with any field, elder abuse prevention has been shaped and defined by a confluence of events, discoveries, and happenstance. Most histories have highlighted milestones in the development of public policy and research. But there are also overarching pressures, forces, and trends that have defined us, shaped the service delivery network, and propelled us in new directions. Some have emerged from within the field, whereas others have been imposed from without.

In this chapter, I have identified eight trends that I believe have particular significance for practice in the field today. Some are related and interconnected, whereas others are in opposition. There are undoubtedly other forces at work as well, but I believe these provide a good starting point for discussing where we have been, where we are now, and where we are going:

1. Increasingly frail elders living at home
2. Shifting paradigms: From protection to empowerment
3. Heightened understanding of victims
4. The circle widens: The burgeoning abuse prevention network
5. The changing role of APS
6. The "criminalization" of elder abuse
7. Focus on forensics
8. Going global: International initiatives to prevent elder abuse

1. INCREASINGLY FRAIL ELDERS LIVING AT HOME

When I started working for the San Francisco Consortium in 1983, it was an exciting time to be in the field of aging. Mount Zion Hospital, where I worked, offered home care, adult day health care, and case management. It was just wrapping up a research and demonstration project that compared the costs and benefits of nursing homes to those of community-based care for frail elders. Within the next few years, half a dozen new programs were launched.

What these programs had in common was the goal of enabling frail elders to live at home. The home-care program brought skilled nursing care into clients' homes, and the adult day health program brought those who would otherwise be relegated to nursing homes to the center, where professionals provided skilled nursing, medical monitoring, and rehabilitative services. Not surprisingly, the research project showed that it was cheaper to keep frail elders at home, up to a certain point at least, when clients' needs became so great that nursing home care made more sense (Miller, Clark, & Clark, 1998). Clients' ability to remain at home depended on case managers who carefully assessed their needs, crafted complicated service plans, arranged for services, and monitored how things were going. Mount Zion was not unique in its preoccupation with keeping clients at home. Agencies around the country were doing the same.

What was remarkable to me was the precariousness of many elderly clients' situations. It was not unusual for the case managers to arrange for attendants to come to clients' homes for an hour or two in the morning to help them get up, dressed, and ready to be picked up and taken to the adult day health care center. There, they would get their only hot meal of the day; have their health status and medications checked; and receive occupational, physical, or speech therapy. Evenings, other attendants might come to help them get ready for bed. A single event like an attendant not showing up for work on time could have a ripple effect, resulting in clients missing meals, treatment, therapy, or medical appointments. It was often a balancing act for their case managers. Two decades earlier, concerns about incapacitated elders and adults with disabilities living alone in the community with nobody to help them had prompted amendments to the Social Security Act, which created an "adult protective services" (APS) safety net. The purpose of APS was to provide legal, social, and support services aimed at preventing institutionalization, abuse, and neglect (Anetzberger, 2005). It was not a perfect system. When I started, there were only two dedicated APS workers in San Francisco and a few workers in other county programs who carried some additional APS cases. Other communities were similarly understaffed.

In light of the situation, it was not surprising that the first early congressional hearings on elder abuse and neglect, which began in 1978, focused on frail elders who depended on others for care. What is often cited as the inaugural step in elder abuse public policy in the United States was testimony before the House of Representatives during a hearing that was attempting to identify the overlooked or ignored aspects of family violence (U.S. House of Representatives, 1978, p. 159). Over the next twenty-five years, many more congressional hearings were held, reports issued, and legislation proposed (Wolf, 2003).

By the late 1980s, it seemed as though we were keeping everyone at home who could reasonably be kept there safely. But later developments suggested otherwise. Foremost among these was the "Olmstead Decision."

In 1995, the Atlanta Legal Aid Society filed *Olmstead v. L. C.* (1999) on behalf of two women who were patients in a state psychiatric hospital. After those treating the women agreed that they could be discharged into community programs, the women were not released until many months later. The court found that the state's failure to release them when it was appropriate to do so was a violation of their civil rights. In essence, the case established community-based care, with reasonable accommodation, as a right protected under the Americans with Disabilities Act. An executive order followed, challenging states to develop more opportunities for people with disabilities to live at home through reforms in health care, transportation, housing, education, and other social supports.

The decision had sweeping impact. States across the country created Olmstead-related task forces to develop plans for making sure that people with disabilities were living in the least restrictive settings possible (Fox-Grage, Coleman, & Folkemer, 2004). The decision also fueled the "consumer-directed care," or "consumer choice," movement, which was aimed at empowering health care "consumers" to exercise greater choice and direct their own care. The Centers for Medicare & Medicaid Services (CMS) awarded millions of dollars in grants for consumer choice programs and the Robert Wood Johnson Foundation has provided additional major funding.

Although consumer choice programs vary, a primary goal is to prevent unnecessary institutionalization. Some programs even assess nursing home patients to determine if they can be transferred into community-based settings. To promote the goal of greater consumer choice, beneficiaries of publicly funded services have been provided with more opportunities to direct their own care. Some, for example, receive vouchers instead of services; the vouchers can be used for home repair or modifications or to purchase assistive devices. Some programs permit consumers to select and manage their own caregivers instead of having licensed home-care professionals do so for them. They may have the option of hiring friends, neighbors, and family members.

Although these developments clearly suggest the need for reinforcing the safety net, state Olmstead plans do not typically address the need for additional protective services. Perhaps more disturbing is the fact that there has been little interaction between the consumer choice and APS or elder abuse prevention networks, and in some instances the two have operated in opposition to each other. For example, many in the field of elder abuse prevention have called for action to reduce the heightened risk of abuse and neglect by independent home-care providers, while consumer choice advocates have argued that consumer-direction programs do not place older adults at heightened risk (Matthias & Benjamin, 2003; Squillace & Firman, 2004).

2. SHIFTING PARADIGMS: FROM PROTECTION TO EMPOWERMENT

The elder abuse prevention field's early focus on protecting frail elders and the patterning of APS on CPS led to frequent charges of ageism and paternalism (Kleinschmidt, 1997; Macolini, 1995). APS professionals have consequently taken pains to distinguish themselves from their colleagues in CPS by emphasizing their commitment to client autonomy, self-determination, and personal freedom (see Chapter 3). They, and others who work with abused and vulnerable elders, have adopted new services and approaches that emphasize empowerment and extended their focus to include elders who are not frail and dependent. In doing so, they have drawn from the fields of domestic violence and victims' rights, adapting techniques like consciousness-raising, options counseling, support groups, safety planning, and legal advocacy (see Chapter 3 for descriptions of these models and Chapter 5 for descriptions of specific services).

This trend is further reflected in the renaming and reframing of public policy related to elder abuse. The labeling of the first comprehensive federal legislation on elder abuse the "Elder Justice Act," for example, emphasizes both societal and personal empowerment for elders. From a societal perspective, vulnerable and abused elders are entitled to parity with respect to services and access to the justice systems. From an individual perspective, elders, including those with diminished capacity, have the right to live free of abuse, neglect, and exploitation, while maintaining their autonomy.

3. HEIGHTENED UNDERSTANDING OF VICTIMS

One of the conundrums of working with abused and vulnerable elders is that many refuse help. Their reticence stems from many factors, including fear of retribution or making matters worse, shame, loyalty to abusers, social and cultural prohibitions, and distrust of the protective service and legal systems.

Professionals in the field responded by writing articles, giving speeches, and organizing training events that focused on "resistant and reluctant" clients. Through these activities, we reminded others and ourselves that our charge was to protect clients' civil liberties as well as their safety. Still, many were uncomfortable with our collective failure to engage clients in the helping process. This frustration may well account for the enthusiasm we have seen for each new discovery or insight that helps explain why clients do what they do and, perhaps more importantly, why they often don't do what we think they should.

There have been several "breakthroughs" that enriched our understanding of victimization, the help-seeking process, and how we can help. The infusion of domestic violence theory, research, and practice into our field, which began in the early 1990s, alerted us to the power and control dynamics operating in some abusive relationships and to the social, economic, and cultural obstacles many victims face. The domestic violence model, which is described in Chapter 3, also acknowledges that violence within relationships does not occur randomly but follows patterns or cycles, which affect victims' receptivity to help and account for the fact that many refuse or change their minds many times before taking decisive action to stop the violence. Understanding that victims march to the beat of their own drums, and that accepting help is a process rather than a single decision, suggested the need for service providers to reevaluate their thinking about how they could help.

Other fields have also shed light on victims, abusers, and the relationships between them and given us new tools. The field of victimology has taught us how to work with people who suffer from post-traumatic stress disorder (PTSD), diminished self-esteem, and isolation; and the field of family caregiver support has helped us understand the dynamics in caregiving relationships and how to intervene when conflicts occur. Neutralization theory, which emerged from the field of criminology, explains how abusers rationalize their behavior and how victims may reinforce these rationalizations. These models and the guidance they offer are described in greater detail in Chapter 3.

Heightened understanding about cognitive functioning and its relationship to decision-making capacity has also helped us better understand and serve elderly victims. Diminished capacity not only increases vulnerability to certain forms of abuse but also may impair elders' ability to understand what has happened, take action to stop abuse, and plan for the future. It further determines what services and interventions are available to them. Whereas capacity was once viewed as a "you've got it or you don't" proposition, we now understand that specific mental skills like memory, the ability to calculate, and orientation to time and place are needed for specific tasks and that some tasks require greater skill than others. We have learned more about how impairments in these areas affect our everyday lives. More recently, we have achieved a clearer understanding of "executive functions," which include complex, subtle mental abilities such as being able to plan for the future or the mental flexibility to shift from one mental task to another. These complex processes further affect elders' ability to act in their own self-interest, protect themselves, or seek or accept help from others. Perhaps nowhere is the research on the psychology of victimization more promising than in the areas of financial abuse and consumer fraud. In recent years, researchers have identified increasingly subtle and complex cognitive deficits, psychological factors, and personality traits that explain why victims fail to recognize seemingly obvious tactics or take steps to protect themselves or seek help. For example, a recent study suggests a link between memory deficit and vulnerability to scams (Jacoby, Bishara, Hessels, & Toth, 2005).

The "discovery" of undue influence as a significant factor in elder abuse further revolutionized thinking, a breakthrough I credit in great part to San Francisco prosecutor Dennis Morris, who came to a meeting of San Francisco's multidisciplinary team over a decade ago and asked the group if anyone knew of an expert in "brainwashing." He was working on a case involving a wealthy woman in her nineties who had recently been spirited off to Nevada for a quickie wedding to a much younger man. The man had moved into the older woman's home and was in the process of appropriating her assets when a relative got suspicious and initiated an investigation. Despite the justice of the peace's assurances that the elderly bride knew what she was doing, Morris was not convinced. Some members of our team found his request a bit odd, as nobody was talking about undue influence in relation to elder abuse back then, but someone suggested he speak to Margaret Singer, a psychologist and expert on cults, brainwashing, and deprogramming prisoners of war.

Morris contacted Singer, who studied the case and subsequently testified before a grand jury. She described the classic forms of social persuasion that the younger man and an accomplice had used to get the older woman to "willingly" allow them to take over her home and property (Nerenberg, 1996). According to Singer, undue influence has little to do with intelligence or cognition, and anyone can be unduly influenced if "artful manipulators," as she called them, are artful enough. To understand the older woman's apparent compliance, Singer explained, examiners needed to look beyond the older woman's mental status at the time she took her vows and consider the psychological manipulations that had been exerted on her prior to the event. This process included isolating her and fostering dependency. They also instilled a "siege mentality," convincing her that the voices she heard coming from outside her house were those of drug dealers and that it was too dangerous for her to go out or let others in. In fact, she lived in one of San Francisco's poshest neighborhoods, and the voices belonged to security guards at a nearby consulate. The perpetrator was convicted in what became a landmark case, and Singer went on to write and lecture extensively about undue influence in elder abuse. Many others followed, enriching our understanding of undue influence.

4. THE CIRCLE WIDENS: THE BURGEONING ABUSE PREVENTION NETWORK

The multidisciplinary nature of elder abuse prevention has long been recognized and is reflected in our research, policy, and practice. State reporting laws enlist the help of professionals from diverse fields to identify cases, multidisciplinary teams have become a hallmark in elder abuse prevention, and diverse groups have received training in abuse detection and response.

The range of disciplines that are acknowledged to have a role in abuse prevention has continually been stretched. Year after year, states have amended their reporting laws to extend coverage to include such far-ranging groups as clergy, employees of financial institutions, and animal care and control workers.

Multidisciplinary teams, which historically included APS workers, mental health professionals, case managers, medical and health care providers, lawyers, police, and many others, have broadened their memberships to include ethicists, judges, clergy, bankers, animal rights advocates, and many more. Beginning in the mid-1990s, new "hybrid" teams began to appear to address specific forms of abuse, bringing even greater diversity to teams (Teaster & Nerenberg, 2003). (See Chapter 6 for more on multidisciplinary teams.) The first Financial Abuse Specialist Team (FAST), started in Los Angeles, brought in stockbrokers, private fiduciaries, bank personnel, experts in insurance and real estate, and many others. Because certain types of financial abuse fall within the jurisdiction of federal law enforcement and regulatory agencies, representatives from U.S. attorneys' offices, the Federal Bureau of Investigation, the Federal Trade Commission, the Secret Service, the Social Security Administration, the Postal Service, and others have joined.

Another new form of hybrid team is the death, or fatality, review team. These teams—which were formed to achieve a clearer understanding of elder deaths, help prosecutors build cases, distinguish "natural" deaths from accidents or homicides, and explore systemic problems or professional conduct that led to deaths—may include coroners, medical examiners, funeral home directors, morticians, hospice care staff, homicide investigators, and others. Medically focused teams, formed to offer increasingly specialized medical assessments, chart reviews, and consultation, may include members with expertise in such areas as geriatrics, forensics, psychiatry, emergency medicine, and others.

The elastic boundaries of the field are further evidenced by the wide range of professionals who have received training in abuse detection and response. Groups for whom training curricula and programs have been developed in recent years include dentists, victim advocates, emergency medical services personnel, bank employees, judges, prosecutors, securities specialists, librarians, sexual assault teams, and many others.

5. THE CHANGING ROLE OF APS

When APS programs first began, workers' primary role was to assess vulnerable adults' need for social and protective services. Later, when states passed reporting laws that made APS responsible for receiving and investigating abuse reports, workers assumed new roles. Whereas APS workers had traditionally focused on clients' social service needs, regardless of what had created those needs, they were increasingly called upon to classify abuse and neglect, substantiate it, and identify perpetrators; and they started working more closely with law enforcement. Over time, as more cases were handled through the criminal and civil justice systems, APS workers began to play an even greater role in collecting evidence, substantiating claims, and testifying in legal proceedings. Some APS units now operate abuse registries, which contain information about offenders that may be used to build legal cases or alert prospective employers.

Even in cases that do not involve perpetrators—when a client's need for help stems from health or mental health problems, lack of resources, or lack of information about or access to resources—workers may feel compelled to categorize situations as "self-abuse" or "self-neglect," suggesting that it is the client who is responsible for his or her circumstances. These heightened pressures to "name and blame" (to label conduct as abuse and identify who is responsible) have created additional challenges.

Often it is not apparent whether neglect is self-imposed or whether others are responsible. Distinguishing neglect from self-neglect may also involve determining whether a client has sufficient capacity to consent to or refuse help, whether the incapacity is permanent, and whether others have a "duty" or responsibility to provide care. While psychologists and legal experts still struggle with these issues, APS workers are forced to make informal judgments about them on a daily basis.

Pressures to name and blame can also have a negative impact on workers' relationships with their clients or even create conflicts of interest. When clients do not want to see their abusers punished, APS workers may find their roles as advocates and investigators incompatible. Workers' role as investigators may alienate clients or destroy their trust in workers. The recent emphasis on identifying abuse and abusers may also distort perceptions about APS. Workers are increasingly viewed by some as quasi law enforcers rather than as service providers whose primary goal is to provide support and services.

The "stakes" for making misjudgments and mistakes with respect to clients' level of risk, to who is responsible, and to appropriate interventions have become much greater. In the early days of APS, when workers simply determined whether someone needed services, they could risk erring on the side of caution. If they wrongly determined that someone was at risk, it simply resulted in that person receiving social and support services he or she was not entitled to. Today, however, when workers conclude that abuse has occurred, it can have extremely negative repercussions for alleged abusers. It may disqualify them from employment or even prompt criminal investigations or civil proceedings. Wrong decisions can expose agencies and individual workers to lawsuits or disciplinary action. To help them function in this new environment, workers are being provided with increasingly complex and sophisticated instruction and instruments, which are described in Chapter 3 (Moskowitz, 1998; Otto, 2000; Roby & Sullivan, 2001).

6. THE "CRIMINALIZATION" OF ELDER ABUSE

One of the most dramatic changes in recent years is the increasing number of elder abuse cases that are being prosecuted. This trend can be credited to the pioneering efforts of creative and tenacious police, prosecutors, and lawmakers who have introduced new techniques, procedures, and statutory innovations (American Prosecutors Research Institute, 2003). These include enhanced penalties for crimes involving elders; "evidence-based prosecution," an approach designed to help prosecutors build cases even when victims are unavailable or unwilling to participate; and specialized elder abuse units within police and prosecutors' offices. Law enforcement officials are increasingly being encouraged to consider domestic violence crimes, when applicable, when charging elder abuse cases.

Criminalizing abuse sends out a clear message to perpetrators that abuse is not tolerated by society; a message that not only is believed to have a deterrent effect but also may further serve to counter the rationalizations that abusers make to themselves and others. (See Chapter 3 under "Neutralization Theory.") It conveys to perpetrators that they must answer not only to victims but also to society, which will bring to bear the resources of the criminal justice system. Incarcerating perpetrators obviously protects victims and potential victims, at least temporarily, and provides supervision and leverage over perpetrators prior to, after, or in lieu of incarceration. Perpetrators can also be ordered to pay restitution to those they have harmed, serve their communities, or undergo treatment.

Along with these benefits, however, come new challenges. The criminal justice system is poorly equipped to handle certain types of elder abuse cases, such as domestic disturbances involving spouses with dementias. In jurisdictions that have mandatory arrest policies for domestic violence, law enforcement officials may feel compelled to make arrests in these cases. Additional problems associated with domestic violence laws are described in greater detail in Chapter 3.

There seems to be a perception among some that criminal justice approaches to elder abuse are in opposition to, or in conflict with, therapeutic or supportive approaches aimed at reinforcing caregiving networks, relieving stress on caregivers, and addressing the social, emotional, and financial needs of family units. This belief may stem from understandable fears that workers will confuse "caregiving issues" with domestic violence, leading to inappropriate responses or even using caregiver stress as an appropriate defense in criminal abuse cases. The 2002 Canadian video *What's Age Got to Do with It* offers a poignant account of what can happen when service providers miss the signs of lethal domestic violence by a caregiver.[1] Although these concerns are understandable, this either-or attitude toward criminal and therapeutic approaches fails to acknowledge the wide variations that characterize elder abuse. It further threatens to polarize the dementia care and criminal justice networks at a time when collaboration is sorely needed to devise effective, humane, and appropriate approaches.

7. FOCUS ON FORENSICS

The focus on holding perpetrators accountable has heightened the need to build legal cases against abusers and highlighted the problems inherent in doing so. Because abuse typically occurs in private and victims are often unable or unwilling to tell outsiders what happened, proving abuse often involves "letting the evidence speak for itself," supplemented by research and expert testimony.

But the evidence in elder abuse cases does not typically speak for itself. Because elders bruise more easily than young people, fall more often, and are more likely to have illnesses and conditions that mimic abuse and neglect, proving abuse often involves demonstrating that injuries were inflicted, not accidental; that neglect was willful, not benign; and that deaths were not "natural" (Dyer, Connolly, & McFeeley, 2003). These challenges have resulted in heightened attention to forensics, which is defined as the "application of science to law." It uses scientific methods to analyze and interpret evidence to determine what happened, when it happened, and whether explanations and defenses are plausible. Medical forensics experts attempt to explain how, when, and why injuries occurred. They draw from forensics medical studies, which explore and compare the "mechanisms" and patterns of inflicted injuries and those of natural occurrence. Other types of forensic experts who may be needed in elder abuse cases include forensics accountants, forensic radiologists (Brogdon, 1998), forensic odontologists (Golden, 2004), forensic entomologists (Benecke, Josephi, & Zweihoff, 2004), forensic psychiatrists (Naimark, 2001), and many more.

Both the federal and state governments have responded to the need for forensics expertise. At the national level, the U.S. Department of Justice (DOJ), in October of 2000, hosted the National Symposium on Forensics Issues in Elder Abuse, a discussion between researchers, medical and forensics experts, and practitioners from the fields of health care, social services, and law enforcement. After reviewing the current state of the art and challenges involved in identifying and substantiating abuse and neglect, the group called for research to establish abuse "markers" (indicators that reliably predict abuse) and other evidence-based data to support findings of abuse, clearinghouses of forensics experts who are available to testify or consult in cases, and databases of documented findings that can be used by prosecutors (Dyer, Pavlik, Murphy, & Hyman, 2003).

Since then, the DOJ has continued to play a leadership role (McNamee & Murphy, 2006). It has supported several studies, including one on bruising at the University of California–Irvine (UCI) that provides baseline data on "natural" bruising that can serve as the basis for evaluating nonnatural bruising (Mosqueda, Burnight, & Liao, 2005). UCI is conducting another study of the rates of pressure ulcers in nursing homes, which will be used to help identify substandard care. Another DOJ-sponsored study examined coroners' reports of elderly nursing home residents in Arkansas to identify abuse markers, and a third explores markers by cross-referencing data on abuse taken from an APS databank in Texas with state medical examiners' reports.

States have also contributed. California supported the development of a forensics assessment tool, enacted legislation allowing elder fatality review teams to share information, and provided technical assistance and training to teams. Local communities and agencies have also gotten involved by organizing death review teams, launching forensics centers, and providing APS programs with access to forensics experts. These state and local initiatives are described in Chapters 6, 7, and 8.

8. GOING GLOBAL: INTERNATIONAL INITIATIVES TO PREVENT ELDER ABUSE

Elder abuse was first recognized in Great Britain, the United States, and Canada; and for many years, most research, program development, and practice emerged from these countries. But in the late 1990s, researchers and service providers from around the world began to meet at international professional conferences to discuss abuse, and, in 1997, a small group launched the International Network for the Prevention of Elder Abuse (INPEA).

Several major developments followed. In 2002, the United Nations (UN) convened the Second World Assembly on Aging in Madrid, Spain. During the event, delegates adopted an International Plan of Action, which acknowledged elder abuse as a human rights and public health issue and included recommendations for addressing it (United Nations Economic and Social Council, 2002). Follow-up activities include the Worldwide Environmental Scan of Elder Abuse, which is being conducted by INPEA in partnership with three universities. Scanning is the identification of emerging issues, events, trends, situations, and potential pitfalls used for planning and decision making. The elder abuse scan is a computerized survey, posted on INPEA's Web site, that solicits information on public policy, services, educational resources, and training on elder abuse. In 2002, the UN's International Research and Training Institute for the Advancement of Women (INSTRAW) sponsored an electronic discussion forum, "Gender Aspects of Violence and Abuse of Older Persons," which drew participants from around the world and highlighted issues of abuse in developing countries (AgeingNet, 2002).

The World Health Organization (WHO) has also called for a world strategy to combat the problem. To learn more about what was needed, WHO collaborated with INPEA, HelpAge International (a global network of nongovernmental, nonprofit organizations, or NGOs), and representatives from academic institutions around the world, in conducting focus groups of elders and primary health care workers[2] in Argentina, Austria, Brazil, Canada, India, Kenya, Lebanon, and Sweden. The focus groups identified key themes, perceptions, beliefs, and attitudes, which are summarized in the report *Missing Voices: Views of Older Persons on Elder Abuse* (WHO/INPEA, 2002).

These initiatives have revealed that elder abuse is defined and perceived very differently around the world. For example, disrespect of elders is viewed as one of the most prevalent and painful forms of abuse. Focus group members in the WHO/INPEA study cited the abandonment of family members in health care facilities such as hospitals as a major problem, with some identifying it as the most frequent form of abuse. Hospital staff in Kenya estimated that between 15% and 30% of older patients end up abandoned in hospitals owing no doubt to the fact that elders or their families have to pay for health care services. Placing elder family members in nursing homes was considered by many respondents to be a form of elder abuse. In the developing countries, placement into long-term care was regarded as a last response for the very poorest people who had no family to care for them.

The "global perspective" on elder abuse attributes abuse and neglect to a variety of factors, many of which reflect underlying economic and social inequalities. The status of elderly women in society is a common theme. A report from the UN secretary-general to the World Assembly on Aging acknowledged the role of sexism and ageism in elder abuse (United Nations Economic and Social Council, 2002), citing "patrilineal inheritance laws and land rights" among the factors that contribute to older women's vulnerability. Participants in the INSTRAW forum further pointed out the futility of addressing elder abuse while ignoring the broader context of institutionalized sexism and ageism that have led to such blatant abuses against women and girls as female feticide (the aborting of female fetuses) and *karo kari* (honor killings), which are still practiced in some developing countries despite efforts to eradicate them (AgeingNet, 2002).

Changing social roles are also blamed. The influx of women worldwide into the job market has reduced the availability of family caregivers, traditionally women, which is believed to result in emotional and physical neglect as well as verbal and physical abuse. The lack of social security systems, fair pensions, and legal protections with respect to inheritance laws also contributes. Worldwide, only 30% of elders are covered by pension plans, leaving many elders without income (United Nations Economic and Social Council, 2002). The situation is worse for women. In many African countries, for example, widows' property is passed on to their elder sons or back to their husbands' families. In other traditional societies, older widows are subject to abandonment and "property grabbing."

Elders' lack of access to health care and social services is another common theme. A decrease in rates of communicable diseases in the developing world over the last few decades has increased the prevalence of long-term, disabling diseases and the need for long-term care. Lack of public funding for basic services puts financial pressure, stress, and burden on families. The poorest members of society are the worst off, and many older adults (especially older women) fall into this category.

Health care professionals are viewed as part of the problem. WHO/INPEA focus group members claimed that health care workers were inadequately trained in aging and older people's problems and did not have enough time to listen to elderly patients. Many, however, view health care providers as victims too, citing poor working conditions and low pay as contributing to abuse. Nurses at one hospital confessed that they "do not look kindly upon older patients who have trouble settling their bills" because they realize that their working conditions will only improve with larger revenues from patients. Others agreed that there was a link between the treatment of workers and the treatment of patients. Many also felt that there was prejudice against geriatrics as a field and that other health care professionals and administrators viewed those who work with elders as less qualified, which accounts for low salaries in this specialty.

Other factors contributing to abuse and neglect that have been identified by global forums include economic crises, the influence of the media in promoting ageist attitudes and negative stereotypes, and westernization. As a result of economic downturns in Argentina and Brazil, for example, adult children are moving back into their parents' homes, sometimes forcing them to move out. In sub-Saharan African countries, including Mozambique, acts of violence against elderly women often stem from accusations of witchcraft connected with unexplained events (WHO/INPEA, 2002). "Mourning rites of passage" for widows in parts of Africa and South Asia can include cruel practices, sexual violence, forced marriages, and eviction from their homes (WHO/INPEA).

An international study of the various forms of domestic violence, including abuse by adult children against their elderly parents, echoes many of these themes and suggests others (Malley-Morrison, 2004). The study, which used a common survey to explore family violence in twenty-four developing and developed countries, also emphasized the role of poverty, economic policies, the status of women, and historical oppression of minority and indigenous groups in family violence. Other contributing factors that were identified included substance abuse, low rates of literacy, laws or customs that permit physical discipline of children, and civil wars.

The emerging literature on global elder abuse also points out how cultural and religious values and traditions mitigate abuse and neglect, and it suggests approaches to abuse prevention (WHO/INPEA). Strong religious dictates to respect and care for older adults, particularly one's parents, have been cited as an important protective factor against abuse; and, in many countries, religious institutions care for destitute elders. WHO/INPEA focus group members in Kenya pointed out that traditional healers, who are key to religious practice and are typically elders, play an important role in society by providing an alternative to the health care system, which is underfunded, inaccessible to those who are poor, and often seen as corrupt.

Focus group participants in the WHO/INPEA study were further asked to suggest ways to stop elder abuse and neglect. Their recommendations included raising awareness, encouraging positive contact between generations, empowering elders to advocate on their own behalf, and providing recreational facilities and opportunities to combat isolation. Solutions to "structural problems" included the strong protective laws and improved health care.

In response, WHO/INPEA has proposed a global strategy that includes the development of a screening and assessment tool for use in primary health care settings, an educational package on elder abuse for primary health care professionals, the development and dissemination of a research methodology kit to study elder abuse, the development of a minimum data set concerning violence and older people, the dissemination of research findings, and a global inventory of good practices.

CONCLUSION

Our field is still very much a work in progress. This chapter has pointed out some of the shifting paradigms and crosscurrents of thought, values, and ideologies that have defined, shaped, and influenced us. These developments further suggest new challenges and opportunities. I will conclude by pointing out a few of these challenges and opportunities, which are described again in greater detail in Chapters 9 and 10.

As we continue to stretch the limits of our community-based long-term care system to "reasonably accommodate" increasingly frail elders, we will need to devote significant resources and attention to reinforcing the protective service safety net. Specific needs that have emerged from the Olmstead decision and the consumer choice movement include the following:

- Mental health professionals to assess when frail elders need decision makers and advocates

- Training for service providers in how to assess capacity for common tasks and to recognize the need for more comprehensive assessment
- Advocates, guardians, or surrogates to act on behalf of those who are incapable of protecting themselves
- Assistance in finding, screening, and supervising independent home-care workers
- Adequate funding for APS and other investigators to monitor those at greatest risk and to respond to complaints of neglect and abuse
- Support services, including more personal care attendants, home-delivered meal programs, transportation, and so on

Ensuring protection for persons with diminished mental capacity is particularly critical and challenging. It will require further exploration into the needs of "unbefriended elders," a term that is increasingly being used to describe elders with diminished mental capacity; who lack friends, surrogates, and advance directives; and who are at risk or in need of services or interventions (Karp & Wood, 2003). At present, few alternatives exist, other than guardianship, for people once they have lost capacity. Less restrictive alternatives are needed for those who are unable to consent to services or medical treatment, hire and supervise helpers, and stop or prevent abuse and neglect.

Recognizing that there are no one-size-fits-all fixes, we need to continue to take a multifaceted approach that holds perpetrators accountable, empowers victims, and ensures the safety, security, and freedom of the most vulnerable.

Holding perpetrators accountable for their actions through criminal justice interventions is imperative, and we must continue to explore new ways to make the criminal justice system more accessible and responsive to elders. We also need to be mindful of the system's pitfalls, monitor its impact, and explore ways to use the leverage the system offers more effectively. Although arrest, incarceration, and court supervision of offenders are powerful tools for stopping abuse, the criminal justice system can achieve other important goals such as compelling offenders to pay back their victims and communities through restitution and community service and providing strong incentives for them to seek treatment.

The emphasis on holding perpetrators accountable, strengthening the criminal justice response, and empowering victims does not preclude offering support and assistance to abusive or high-risk caregivers, nor does it diminish the importance of social services, treatment, and protection for victims. New discoveries about the psychology of victimization suggest a wide range of interventions that hold promise for overcoming social barriers, psychological manipulation, and intergenerational and long-standing family conflicts.

As the field evolves, we will need to continue to examine, clarify, and define APS workers' role and the viability of workers serving as both investigators and victim advocates. As the consequences of abuse become more severe, as the punishments for abusers increase, and as the repercussions of inaccurate assessments intensify, APS' role will come under increasing scrutiny and perhaps force us to reassess old assumptions.

Finally, there is much to gain from looking beyond our borders for new approaches and perspectives. This is particularly crucial in light of the fact that by 2025, the global population of people over the age of sixty is expected to reach 1.2 billion. One million people turn sixty every month, and 80% of these are in the developing world (WHO/INPEA, 2002). In addition, many of the themes raised in the international literature on elder abuse have been echoed by underserved and disenfranchised groups within wealthier countries. These include the necessity of viewing elder abuse within a broader social, political, and economic context and calling for holistic and integrated approaches that address the needs of families, extended families, cultural groups, and the broader community.

These challenges are formidable. Meeting them will require us to resolve the conflicts that have placed us in opposition to those whose approaches differ from ours. It will require broadening society's perspective on civil rights and liberties to encompass the full life span and exploring ways to ensure the rights and protection of people with diminished capacity. It means working with other advocates, including proponents of consumer choice, to explore ways to preserve independence and autonomy that do not pose unacceptable and needless risks. Just as we have expanded our network to include an ever-widening array of service providers, we need to extend our advocacy network. Failure to do so will lead to counterproductive battles, a lack of unity, incoherent policy, and missed opportunities.

NOTES

1. The video, which was written and directed by Hilary Pryor and produced by The May Street Group Film, is available from Terra Nova Films. For more information, see http://www.terranova.org/SearchResult.aspx?ListType=Title&IDValue=W.

2. In developing countries, the term *primary health care workers* typically refers to nonphysicians, ranging from medical assistants and nurse practitioners to village "mobilizers," volunteers, or aides who combine modern health science and technology with traditional healing to address such basic health issues as family planning, pre- and postnatal care, nutrition, immunization, safe water, basic sanitation, and disease prevention. Most primary health care workers are women and are chosen with input from their communities.

CHAPTER TWO

Defining Elder Abuse: The Controversies

INTRODUCTION

Many years ago, a prominent gerontologist suggested to the audience at a conference I attended that elder abuse was a nonproblem dreamed up by social workers to create jobs for themselves. He went on to say that if society's systems of protection—our social service, legal, and health care systems—were failing to protect elders, they needed to be fixed, not replaced by new systems and bureaucracies.

His cantankerous remarks were clearly intended to spark debate. But over the years, I have given a lot of thought to the fundamental questions the speaker was alluding to: "What sets elder abuse apart from other categories of crime or mistreatment?" and "Do we really need a whole new system to respond?" Two decades have passed since then, and I still do not think our field has come up with an adequate response.

Our collective failure to answer these very basic questions is reflected in the definitional inconsistencies that pervade our literature, public policies, and programs (Daly & Jogerst, 2001). Just about every article ever written or paper presented on elder abuse begins with apologies and caveats for the widely divergent and often conflicting statistics, profiles, and risk factors we offer. We attribute these inconsistencies, to a great extent, to differences in how abuse is defined. Our field's inability to agree on definitions has confounded and riled policy makers, the media, and professionals, and it impedes our ability to develop comprehensive responses.

The responsibility for defining abuse has rested mainly with researchers and policy makers. Those who design and provide services have largely been on the receiving end, using definitions created by others.

I believe that practitioners need to join the definitional debates. Many, I'm sure, will be loathe to do so. Researchers and policy makers spend hours arguing over the inclusion, placement, and nuances of words. But this apparent fixation on semantics and grammar is not gratuitous. The outcome of these discussions has critical implications for practice. For example, the presence of the single word *willful* in front of *abuse* or *neglect* in reporting statutes means that responders only need to concern themselves (theoretically, at least) with cases that involve deliberate or malevolent conduct. It relieves them (again, theoretically) from having to act when abuse or neglect stem from ignorance, exhaustion, lack of resources, mental illness, or dementia. In essence, definitions determine whom practitioners serve, the size of their caseloads, what services are needed, and the resources required to provide them.

Some of the variations in how abuse and neglect are defined are straightforward, and their impact on practice is relatively easy to predict. For example, laws that define *elder* as anyone aged sixty and over will generate more reports than those that use anyone aged sixty-two or sixty-five and over, and clients will be less likely to have age-related impairments. But other differences raise perplexing theoretical and practical questions.

This chapter describes some of the overarching issues, differences, and controversies in defining elder abuse and neglect in general. It then describes the problems and issues involved in defining specific forms. It does not attempt to resolve conflicts, but rather, to shed light on areas of disagreement and highlight their repercussions for practice.

Overarching differences, issues, and controversies regarding definitions of abuse and neglect include:

- Whether it is necessary for elderly victims to have physical and/or mental impairments
- Whether they must be in "special relationships" with their abusers
- Whether the abuse has to be intentional
- Whether abuse and neglect are defined by deeds and conduct, or their impact
- Whether abuse and neglect reflect patterns of conduct (as opposed to single acts)

CONTROVERSIES IN DEFINING ELDER ABUSE

The Disability Requirement

Some believe that what distinguishes elder abuse from other forms of crime or misconduct against elders is the victims' *vulnerability* or *dependence*. These terms refer to the presence of debilitating illnesses or conditions that compromise independence and judgment, and include cognitive, physical, and communication deficits. According to this point of view, elders need special protections because they are likely to have conditions that make them dependent or vulnerable. People who argue for the inclusion of the vulnerability/dependency requirement assume that elders who are healthy and capable have access to traditional, "mainstream" protections and do not, therefore, need specialized services.

State reporting laws vary with respect to vulnerability or dependency requirements (American Prosecutors Research Institute, 2003). Some laws only protect people who are both elderly *and* vulnerable or dependent, whereas other laws apply to all victims over a certain age (usually sixty five). Still others use vulnerability or dependency in lieu of age as the primary criteria for protection (in other words, any abused adult, eighteen years or older, who has mental or physical vulnerabilities, is protected).

What implications does this requirement have for practice? Clearly, programs and agencies that limit coverage to persons who are vulnerable or dependent have to devise methods to screen out the ineligible. Although that may sound straightforward, in practice, it often is not. Deficits that make people vulnerable and dependent may be extremely subtle, and changes may occur gradually. Because comprehensive assessments are costly and labor intensive, agencies rely on simple screening tools like the Mini Mental State Exam (see Chapter 5), which have been widely criticized.

Offering protective services to all abused, neglected, or high-risk adults over a certain age eliminates the costs and uncertainties associated with screening. It does, however, require agencies to serve nonvulnerable, nondependent elderly victims as well as those who are vunerable or dependent.

Who are these able-bodied, elderly victims, and what services do they need? We do not really know because there have not been any systematic analyses. However, APS colleagues in states like California that do not use the dependency criteria report that the able-bodied, independent elders they serve primarily comprise elderly victims of domestic violence, elders who are abused by family members with substance abuse or mental health problems, and victims of fraud.

The "Special Relationship" Requirement

Some definitions of elder abuse stipulate that abusers must be in "special relationships with," or in "positions of trust, confidence, or dependency toward," their victims. This includes family members, friends, acquaintances, caregivers, roommates, intimate partners, service providers, fiduciaries, or anyone who has a financial or legal responsibility toward the victim. These requirements distinguish elder abuse from "stranger crimes," which include street crime or consumer fraud.

In general, crimes and abuse against elders by strangers are excluded from elder abuse definitions and laws, ostensibly because victims are already covered by existing criminal statutes or served by mainstream victim services (Kapp, 1995). The "special relationship" criterion has, however, been revisited in recent years due in part to the fact that the lines between abusers who are strangers and those in special relationships are often blurred. In recent years, for example, we have started to recognize that some predators seek out victims and establish relationships of trust and confidence with the intent of abusing them. Few would argue that strangers who identify grieving widows and widowers through newspaper death announcements or befriend vulnerable elders in supermarket parking lots, and then use the trust they have cultivated to their advantage are guilty of elder abuse. But many draw the line at including perpetrators who contact elders by phone or computer. Emerging research and practice experience, however, suggests that distant and even "virtual" strangers may also establish relationships of trust, confidence, and intimacy. I have provided examples in later sections.

Intentionality

Some definitions of abuse and neglect specify that the conduct must be willful, deliberate, or malicious, thereby excluding abuse and neglect that is unintentional, benign, passive, or the result of recklessness. The "intent requirement" further eliminates abusive conduct committed by persons with mental illnesses, deliriums, developmental disabilities, or dementias, who are considered to be incapable of intent.

Determining whether acts were willful or intentional can be extremely difficult or impossible because it involves "getting inside the heads" of abusers to discover motives, beliefs, perceptions, and intentions. In some situations, it may not even be clear to abusers if their acts were willful or intentional.

Whether or not intent is required depends, to some extent, on the setting and circumstances. For example, the criminal justice system requires a showing of intent to prove certain crimes. On the other hand, social service programs have traditionally focused on victims' needs rather than abusers' motives and attitudes. Even within the social service arena, however, perpetrators' motives, intents, and willingness to change are taken into account because they may have significant repercussions for practice. A frightened, remorseful caregiver who has struck an impaired elder out of desperation or in self-defense may willingly agree to counseling, respite, or instruction. These services may be all that's needed to solve the problem. But when abuse and neglect are motivated by malevolence or greed (e.g., a caregiver wants to hasten an elder's death because he or she is a beneficiary), very different interventions are called for such as arrest, termination from employment, or financial penalties.

Focusing on Conduct or Its Impact

Should elder abuse be defined by the acts or conduct of an abuser, or by the impact of the acts or conduct? Clearly, the impact of physical violence, neglect, and other mistreatment is likely to be greater on elders than younger victims. A hit, a shove, or a push, which may have no lasting impact on a young person, can be devastating to some elders. Owing to these differences, some definitions focus on the impact of acts or conduct instead of, or in addition to, the acts themselves. For example, some define physical abuse as "the use of physical force *that results in injury, physical pain, or impairment.*" Others have expanded the definition further to include conduct that *could* (potentially) cause harm (e.g., "the use of physical force that *may* result in bodily injury, physical pain, or impairment" or "actions that *create a serious risk of harm*"). In contrast, definitions of financial abuse typically focus on the acts rather than their impact.

Frequency and Severity

Some definitions of abuse cover single harmful acts, whereas others require that abuse or neglect be recurrent or ongoing. The number of events or duration required to constitute a pattern of abuse or neglect also varies. Definitions used by researchers that focus on impact may even set very specific thresholds of *lethality,* a term that refers to the extent and seriousness of injury.

WHAT THE EXPERTS SAY

Where do the experts stand on definitions? A panel of researchers and practitioners convened by the National Academy of Sciences (NAS) in

2002 to review and evaluate the research on elder mistreatment adopted a relatively precise and narrow definition:

> (a) Intentional actions that cause harm or create a serious risk of harm (whether or not harm is intended) to a vulnerable elder by a caregiver or other person who stands in a trust relationship to the elder, or (b) failure by a caregiver to satisfy the elder's basic needs or to protect the elder from harm. (National Research Council, 2003)

In defining abuse this way, the NAS panel focused its discussion on intentional conduct, thereby eliminating inadvertent, unintended, or reckless acts. It further excludes acts by people with impairments that render them incapable of intent. It also specifies that there must be a perpetrator (eliminating self-neglect, which is discussed later) and that perpetrators must be in special relationships toward their victims, which eliminates abuse by strangers. The inclusion of the word *vulnerable* can be taken to mean that abuse against able-bodied elders is not included.

In contrast, the Elder Justice Act uses a very sketchy definition of abuse:

> The knowing infliction of physical or psychological harm or the knowing deprivation of goods or services that are necessary to meet essential needs or to avoid physical or psychological harm.

In adopting this definition, legislators avoided the thorny questions of whether to include vulnerability as a prerequisite for protection, relationships between victims and abusers, and thresholds of frequency and severity. The term *knowing* suggests that abuse must be intentional although it is not explicit. Because this definition will determine the number of elders who are entitled to protection, the services they will need, and the costs of providing them these services, it is clear that this definition will be hotly debated in the future.

CHALLENGES IN DEFINING SPECIFIC FORMS OF ABUSE

In addition to these overarching issues and controversies, defining specific forms of abuse pose additional, unique challenges. In this section, definitions of the various forms of abuse used by the National Center on Elder Abuse are presented, followed by a brief discussion of additional concerns that each raises.

Financial Abuse

Financial abuse encompasses a wide range of conduct. It includes personal care attendants shortchanging elderly clients; children assuming control over their parents' homes or property for their own benefit; predatory lenders misleading older homeowners into taking out home equity loans they cannot pay back; "sweetheart scammers" courting elders with the intent of defrauding them; and family members with substance addictions taking money or property to support their habits.

Controversies about how to define financial abuse go back many years. An early Delphi survey of experts addressed the issue of whether financial abuse should include abuse by professional fiduciaries, bankers, and other professionals, as well as abuse by family members and acquaintances. The experts agreed the definition should include abuse by these professionals (Johnson, 1986).

Defining what constitutes "special relationships" or "positions of trust and confidence" with respect to financial abuse can be complicated. As mentioned earlier, the boundaries between strangers and people in positions of trust and confidence may be unclear because financial predators often start out as strangers but establish relationships of trust with their victims. In doing so, they use a wide array of "influence" tactics matching their pitches to the psychological needs of their victims.

Although most in our field would consider the situations just described to be elder financial abuse, many draw the line at including telemarketing fraud, predatory lending, and identity theft. Yet today, cunning predators operating out of Canada, Africa, or Europe are increasingly using the phone or Internet to gain their victims' trust and confidence, calling daily or multiple times a day, sending greeting cards, telling them bogus hard-luck stories that are accompanied by requests for money, and even making romantic overtures (Deem, Nerenberg, & Titus, 2007).

Another perceived stranger crime is identity theft. Although it has rarely been included in definitions of elder abuse, recent studies suggest that this form of abuse is most often committed by family members, acquaintances, and employees (Javelin Strategy and Research, 2005). In particular, identity theft by personal care attendants and nursing home employees is increasingly being reported.

In addition to these "special relationship" requirements, definitions of financial abuse have traditionally tended to emphasize cognitive impairment. In fact, cognitive impairment is a prerequisite or primary risk factor for certain forms of financial abuse (Heath, Brown, Kobylarz, & Castaño, 2005). For example, inducing someone who is incapable of exercising informed consent to enter into a financial agreement can itself be considered a form of financial abuse.

The focus on cognitive impairment in financial abuse is another reason that telemarketing and other "consumer" crimes are left out of abuse definitions. That is because some studies have shown that victims of these crimes are no more likely than nonvictims to have cognitive impairments

(AARP, 1996). The emerging literature on fraud, however, suggests that victims of certain frauds are likely to have very subtle cognitive impairments that account for their failure to recognize seemingly obvious tactics or take steps to protect themselves or seek help. For example, a recent study suggests a link between memory deficit and vulnerability to scams (Jacoby, Bishara, Hessels, & Toth, 2005).

Insisting that definitions of financial abuse include the requirement that victims have cognitive impairments may make sense from a theoretical perspective because those who are not impaired have access to traditional protections such as the criminal and civil justice systems. In practice, however, determining whether someone has a cognitive impairment that places him or her at risk of financial abuse is extremely complicated as these deficits may be extremely subtle. In addition, elders may be financially abused in many ways using a wide array of legal and financial instruments such as powers of attorney, trusts, guardianships, annuities, and so on. The requisite capacity for various financial and legal instruments, transactions, and decisions also vary widely. And, although capacity for certain actions is relatively easy to assess and there is agreement on what criteria or measures to use, others are highly complex and controversial.

Unlike definitions of physical abuse, which are likely to focus on the harm caused or the potential for harm, definitions of financial abuse tend to focus on the actual conduct rather than its impact. They do not typically specify, for example, that the conduct must result in hardship or loss. Similarly, most definitions do not take into account the fact that a relatively small loss can be devastating to elders with limited assets and on fixed incomes, whereas much larger losses may have less impact on wealthier people. Although these differences are not typically reflected in definitions, they are sometimes acknowledged in practice. Some prosecutors, for example, have lowered the monetary threshold they use in deciding what elder abuse cases to take.

Physical Abuse

Physical abuse encompasses a wide range of conduct, from single acts of violence, which may or may not cause serious harm, to escalating violence that has gone on for many years. As described earlier, definitions of physical abuse have traditionally focused on the impact of the abusive acts or conduct, or the potential impact. Although not explicitly stated in definitions, physical abuse has generally been taken to mean abuse by persons in special relationships toward their victims including spouses, sons and daughters, and caregivers. Assaults by strangers have not traditionally been included.

In the last fifteen years, particular attention has been paid to several subsets of physical abuse, including elder domestic violence, elder homicide, and elder suicide/homicide. Elder domestic violence has been of particular interest, although the definitions that are used vary widely. The lack of agreement surrounding these definitions reflects broader controversies regarding how domestic violence in general is or should be defined (these changes and controversies are described in Chapter 3). Historically, domestic violence was defined as an on-going and escalating pattern of violence and intimidation committed by males against female intimate partners for the purpose of gaining power and control. Power and control was rooted in men's privileged status in society. This definition was similarly applied to elder domestic violence in the early literature on the subject. (For more on domestic violence, see Chapter 3.)

Today, however, the term *domestic violence* may refer to a wider range of conduct. It may include violence by women against men, violence within same-sex intimate relationships, and violence by nonintimate family members, including sons and daughters. The requirements that violence be repetitive, escalating, or related to gender or social inequality have been removed from many definitions. New definitions such as *intimate partner violence, gender-based violence,* and *violence against women* have emerged to highlight specific forms or attributes of violence and lend greater clarity.

Many in our field acknowledge the existence of several subcategories of elder domestic violence (Seaver, 1996). These include "domestic violence grown old," which refers to violence that began earlier and continues into old age, and "late-onset" domestic violence, which refers to domestic violence that starts or worsens in later life. Older women may also enter into new, abusive relationships in later life.

Other patterns that practitioners have observed include *dementia-related domestic violence* and *reverse domestic violence,* which refers to the fact that some elderly victims retaliate against abusive partners who have become debilitated. There is, however, little agreement about the validity or usefulness of these terms. In the case of dementia-related violence, the element of power and control, one of the few elements of domestic violence for which there is still widespread agreement, may not be present.

The emergence of "elder domestic violence" as a subcategory of elder abuse poses new challenges. The changing and inconsistent definitions of domestic violence that are currently in use contribute to and compound the problems that already exist in defining elder abuse. This lack of clarity has potentially serious consequences such as subjecting parties in elder abuse cases to inappropriate interventions. For example, in jurisdictions that have mandatory arrest policies for domestic violence, law enforcement officials may feel compelled to take violent spouses, intimate partners, or adult children into custody even if their conduct results from dementia or mental illness.

Although seldom defined, the terms "gray death," "elder homicides," and "elder murders" are generally applied to inflicted deaths that were concealed or made to look like natural deaths (Collins & Presnell, 2006). They typically involve strangulation, which may leave no apparent injuries, poisoning using common prescription medications, or claims that deaths resulted from accidents or suicides. As these cases become more common, more precise definitions and distinctions will clearly be needed.

Finally, the relatively new subcategory of elder homicide-suicide emerged when researchers in Florida who were studying what they originally thought were "double suicides" discovered that, in some cases, one partner was not a willing participant. The nonconsensual nature of these acts was evidenced by defensive wounds indicating that one partner had fought back or a lack of evidence suggesting that one partner was suicidal (Cohen, 2000). In some of the cases, there had been a history of domestic violence. Others involved "dependent protective" long-term relationships, in which one partner (most often the man) dominated (Cohen, 2000).

Elder Sexual Abuse

Elder sexual abuse includes violent sexual acts such as rape and sodomy, molestation, and sexual acts with people who are incapable of consenting as a result of cognitive or communication impairments. Nonviolent sexual abuse also includes sexual harassment such as being forced to listen to or watch sexual acts, pornography, or exhibitionism.

Defining sexual assault, whether physically violent or not, is extremely complex for several reasons. Although it is generally agreed that any sexual contact with people who are incapable of consenting as a result of cognitive or communication impairments constitutes sexual abuse, determining if someone is capable of exercising consent to sexual contact is not easy. It is complicated by the fact that individuals who lack capacity to consent may willingly agree to, or even initiate, sexual contact. Culpability in sexual abuse further depends on the perpetrators' knowledge that elders lack the capacity to consent. But determining what abusers knew or should have known with respect to elders' capacity is virtually impossible in many cases.

The relationships between the parties also need to be considered. Clearly, when a spouse or intimate partner initiates sexual contact with an incapacitated elder, it should not be treated the same as sexual contact by strangers. Sexualized touching of an impaired elder by a spouse may provide comfort, pleasure, or reassurance, whereas the same behavior by a stranger constitutes molestation (Lingler, 2003). However, there has been little discussion about when sexual conduct between intimates, when one or both partner is impaired, becomes inappropriate, abusive, or criminal (Jeary, 2004).

These issues related to sexuality among persons with cognitive impairments are not new and have been addressed by personnel in nursing homes, dementia care programs, and other settings for many years. But as awareness about elder abuse increases, it becomes more likely that domestic violence, spousal rape, and sexual assault laws will be invoked in elder abuse cases, thereby calling for greater clarity and consensus with respect to what constitutes elder sexual abuse.

Emotional Abuse

Emotional abuse, also frequently called psychological or verbal abuse, includes threatening, humiliating, ridiculing, cursing, isolating, or infantilizing elders. One of the most challenging aspects of defining and addressing emotional abuse is its highly subjective nature. What can be extremely damaging to one person may not affect someone else. Cultural factors also play a role. Studies show, for example, that within certain cultures, isolation, silence, and verbal abuse are viewed much more seriously than in others (Anetzberger, 1997; Moon et al., 1998; Patterson & Malley-Morrison, 2004). This subjective aspect suggests that definitions should focus on impact as opposed to the acts themselves, which they typically do.

In recent years, attention has been paid to certain forms of psychological abuse, including stalking and pet abuse. Recent research shows that elderly women are almost as likely as younger women to experience stalking, which includes such fear-inducing behavior as vandalizing or burglarizing homes, following someone, threatening to harm them, threatening to harm their loved ones or pets, leaving disturbing telephone or email messages, waiting outside their homes, or sending cards or gifts (Jasinski & Dietz, 2003). Stalking may also be a precursor of domestic violence. Abuse of elders' pets or threats of abuse, which are also increasingly being reported, have also been shown to be correlated with subsequent acts of domestic violence (Humane Society of the United States, n.d.).

Neglect

Neglect includes caregivers' failure to provide necessary treatment, assistance, services, and basic necessities such as medical and mental health care, assistance with bathing and toileting, personal hygiene, food and water, and protection against safety hazards. Neglect is typically defined as a continuing course of conduct; single acts or omissions are typically not seen as neglect (Myers, 2005). This is despite the fact that a single act of serious negligence can be lethal.

Definitions of neglect, like NCEA's above, assume that caregivers have a duty or obligation to provide care, and one of the unique challenges involved in defining and diagnosing this form of abuse is determining who, if anyone, has that duty or responsibility. It may be created by contractual arrangement (the person is paid), assumed voluntarily, or it may arise out of special relationships (e.g., children, spouses).

The extent to which family members are legally responsible to provide care and the type of care required has not been clearly established and varies by state (Moskowitz, 2001). For example, in some states, including Massachusetts and North Carolina, anyone over the age of eighteen who has sufficient means but neglects or refuses to support a parent who is unable to support him/herself due to age or disability is subject to a fine or imprisonment, and, in some jurisdictions, adult children have a duty to provide for their indigent parents to the extent that they are able (National Center for Victims of Crime, 1999). The duty to provide care is also being determined by courts. For example, courts have determined that people have a duty to provide care to spouses who are incapable of deciding whether or not they need help (Payne, 2003). And, in a precedent-setting case, the California Supreme Court determined that an adult child is only criminally liable for a parent's care where the duty is "affirmatively accepted" (*People v. Heitzman*, 1994).

In addition to raising questions about caregivers' responsibilities toward those they care for, defining and diagnosing neglect raises questions about the level of care that is required, expected, or reasonable. The standard that is typically used is what a "reasonable person would provide under like circumstances."

Another controversy related to neglect is whether or not to include the requirement that it be intentional. The terms *passive neglect* and *benign neglect*, which appear in the literature, suggest that neglect may be inadvertent. Unintentional neglect also includes failure to provide care that results from caregivers' lack of physical strength, stamina, emotional stability, maturity, or skills. These forms of neglect are in contrast to "active," willful, or intentional neglect, which may be motivated by malevolence or greed (e.g., when caregivers withhold care in an attempt to hasten elders' death because they stand to inherit).

Neglect is sometimes defined as "an act of omission" rather than commission. This characterization is misleading and potentially damaging because it tends to cast neglect in a less serious light than other forms of abuse when, in fact, neglect can have extremely damaging, life-threatening, or lethal consequences.

Self-Neglect

The terms *abuse* and *mistreatment* typically conjure up images of people doing things to, or not doing things for, others. In contrast, self-neglect refers to people's failure to satisfy their own needs for medical attention, adequate food, self-care, and protection.

There is disagreement as to whether self-neglect should, in fact, be considered a form of abuse and be included in mandatory reporting statutes, other policy, or research studies on elder abuse. Clearly, it adds another layer of vagueness and ambiguity to an already poorly defined problem. As one researcher points out, "The study of self-neglect has been hampered by inadequate conceptualization and a lack of theoretical frameworks" (Lauder, 1999). Those who reject its inclusion point out that self-neglect is really a different problem altogether. It has frequently been described as a mental health problem associated with alcoholism, depression, dementia, and mental illness (Duke, 1991; Dyer, Pavlik, Murphy, & Hyman, 2000; National Research Council, 2003). Self-neglect may also be a symptom of trauma. Because it is more common than any other single form of abuse or neglect by others, its inclusion in research studies and reporting tallies can significantly skew the results.

It is further marred by internal contradictions or inconsistencies. For example, researchers have observed that the majority of self-neglectors are cognitively impaired, which suggests that their ability to exercise choice may be compromised, casting doubt on their ability to consent to (or conversely, withhold consent for) needed care. But the term *self-neglect* is also often applied to elders who are capable of exercising consent to help but refuse to do so. These two situations call for very different responses. If self-neglecting elders lack capacity, involuntary measures are appropriate. On the other hand, if capable clients refuse help, interventions may focus on motivating them to accept help. Ultimately, however, if capable people continue to refuse help, workers must respect their wishes.

The lack of clarity that exists with respect to self-neglect has resulted in the term becoming a "default" for conduct that does not fit neatly into other categories. In addition, a variety of conditions or situations are frequently mistaken for self-neglect, including poverty, eccentricity, and unconventional lifestyles. The term may further be seen as judgmental and stigmatizing because it suggests failure on the part of people to take care of themselves, when, in fact, they have no control over their conduct or situations.

If the conceptual reasons for including self-neglect in definitions of elder abuse are questionable, they may be overshadowed by practical considerations. For example, neglect and self-neglect may be indistinguishable to first responders and other observers who play a key role in making referrals to APS and other agencies that can help. The signs and symptoms are virtually the same and include pressure ulcers, debilitated homes, filth, malnutrition, and general decline. Emergency medical personnel, police, medical professionals, and others who are likely to observe these conditions rarely have the information, time, or skills required to determine if these conditions are self-imposed or the fault of others. They may be reluctant to report situations for fear of incriminating innocent caregivers, jeopardizing their relationships with elders or caregivers, and exposing their agencies to liability. By including self-neglect in reporting laws, responders do not have to distinguish it from neglect by others, which may, therefore, encourage them to report.

Some who support the inclusion of self-neglect in elder abuse reporting laws point out that it is the most common reason for APS referrals (it is estimated to comprise one to two-thirds of APS caseloads) and that including it has elevated its visibility by capitalizing on recent interest in elder abuse. Conversely, if eliminated from definitions, self-neglect might be overshadowed by neglect and abuse by others. On the other hand, removing self-neglect from definitions of elder abuse and addressing it as a separate entity could potentially serve to highlight it as a discrete and unique phenomenon and focus attention on its salient features, including its relationship to declining health status, dementia, substance abuse, depression, recent losses, and trauma.

Abandonment

Abandonment includes leaving elders unattended in public settings, hospital emergency rooms, or in long-term care facilities. Caregivers may leave elders alone without adequate provisions for extended periods, move away, or quit without arranging for substitutes. Abandonment is sometimes defined as a type or symptom of neglect, and the two have features in common. Like neglect, abandonment assumes that perpetrators have a responsibility toward the elders by virtue of being family members or paid caregivers. And, like neglect, it too may be financially motivated. For example, families may take over elders' assets after leaving them in long-term care facilities. Generally, the criterion used to determine whether a caregiver has abandoned an elder is the same standard used for neglect—that is, "what a reasonable person under like circumstances would do." Unlike neglect, which may or may not be willful, abandonment typically refers to willful conduct.

Other

Other forms of elder abuse and neglect sometimes appear in the literature and in reporting laws. These include *violation of rights*, which includes the right to privacy, confidentiality, free choice, religious freedom, freedom to associate with whomever one chooses, freedom to refuse psychotropic medications, and freedom from confinement in locked facilities. Furthermore, individuals in long-term care facilities have the right to medical services, the right to choose physicians, the right to remain in the facility, and freedom from physical restraint or involuntary seclusion.

Abduction includes taking elders from their residences and preventing them from returning through force, coercion, or undue influence. The elder may lack sufficient mental capacity to consent to these moves, and/or the person removing them may lack authority to do so. Elders may be abducted to give perpetrators access to their homes or finances.

Abuse that occurs in long-term care facilities is defined by some as a specific form or category of elder abuse, whereas others view it simply as a setting in which abuse takes place. Those who argue for its inclusion as a separate category of elder abuse and neglect point to its distinctive features and the need for very different responses.

Institutional settings include skilled nursing facilities, intermediate care facilities, assisted living homes, and others. Institutional abuse and neglect typically refer to ongoing patterns of conduct, including chronic neglect, the illegal use of restraints, substandard care, and higher than acceptable rates of falls, pressure ulcers, accidents, and deaths. Institutional abuse also includes negligent or corrupt management practices, such as profiteering, falsifying records to hide mistakes or to make it look like services were provided that were not, failure to provide adequate screening or supervision of staff, and failure to report or respond to problems. In addition, this form of abuse includes failure to protect residents from abusive workers, residents, or visitors. Abuse in institutions may, however, also include individual or repeated acts by direct service staff, family members, guests, visitors, other residents, supervisors, managers, directors, and corporate entities.

The inclusion of abuse and neglect in institutional settings in definitions of elder abuse has already had a critical impact on practice. Police, APS, long-term care ombudsmen, and others have become increasingly involved in investigating and responding to abuse and neglect in facilities. To continue to do so effectively, they will need clearer and consistent definitions.

CONCLUSION

It would be gratifying to conclude this chapter by proposing a definition that would settle the debates once and for all, one that lawmakers, practitioners, and researchers alike would hail as the *definitive* definition of elder abuse. Unfortunately, uniform definitions require agreement on fundamental issues that our field has yet to agree on, or even to discuss seriously.

The fact of the matter is that, in practice, consistency in definitions is neither possible nor desirable. We need different definitions for different settings and purposes. The definitions used to determine eligibility for protective services, for example, should be inclusive enough to capture situations in which there is a high risk of abuse, whereas the definitions used by the criminal justice system should be narrow enough to exclude cases that do not rise to the level of criminal activity.

Although we may never reach consensus, it is important that we move the definitional debate forward. That includes exploring the issues raised in this chapter with respect to how definitions dictate whom we serve, what services they need, and the resources required to do so. Addressing these supply and demand issues is critical for effective advocacy. It is easy for policy makers to turn down funding requests or steer clear of the issue altogether when we cannot agree on fundamental needs.

These discussions need to take place on many levels. But, most importantly, service providers need to be involved. Their perspectives, knowledge, and insights can help policy makers and researchers understand how the definitions translate to the world of clients and services. That input is critical to designing comprehensive services, coherent policy, and practice-focused research that will help serve clients more effectively.

This chapter has identified key controversies that need to be addressed in defining abuse and neglect. Some will be fleshed out in later chapters. Chapter 9, for example, describes the need for research to shed light on how definitions impact the supply and demand for services.

CHAPTER THREE

Service Models from Which We Have Drawn

INTRODUCTION

Program developers in the field of elder abuser prevention have taken an improvisational approach to crafting services and interventions. In doing so, they have recycled, refined, and rejected elements from many service delivery models to produce a rich, if somewhat discordant, mélange.

This chapter describes eight of these models, which span a broad spectrum in terms of origin, ideology, and approach. Adult protective services (APS), the predominant model in the field today, is described first, followed by the domestic violence prevention and public health models, which have both gained prominence in the last few years. The models that follow are less well known perhaps within our field and are presented to draw attention to the promising features they offer.

The models have both common and distinctive features. The domestic violence, victim advocacy, and family caregiver support models, for example, were all products of grassroots advocacy movements that emerged from the social activism of the 1960s and 1970s, whereas it was professionals who advanced the APS and public health approaches. The models also differ in terms of their focus, with neutralization theory concentrating on abusers; the victim advocacy and domestic violence models, on victims; the family caregiver support and family preservation models, on families; and the public health model, on whole communities.

Although other models appear in the elder abuse literature, most of them attempt to explain why abuse occurs and who is at risk. The eight included here were selected because they offer promising approaches to practice. I have briefly described the origins of each, their guiding principles,

35

the services and interventions they offer, what is known about their effectiveness, how they have been applied to elder abuse prevention, and their benefits and limitations.

I am not endorsing or recommending these models. Instead, they are presented to enhance readers' repertoires of skills and to suggest new approaches for agencies, local communities, and states to explore. Hopefully, this chapter will foster a greater appreciation for our field's diversity and versatility, enhance understanding of diverse perspectives, and lead to greater interdisciplinary exchange and collaboration. I am also hoping that it will illustrate the need for, and perhaps point the way toward, a new approach that reflects the unique experiences and diverse needs of vulnerable elders—a model that is uniquely our own.

THE ADULT PROTECTIVE SERVICES (APS) MODEL

Adult Protective Services, the cornerstone of elder abuse prevention in the United States today, actually reflects the fusing of two approaches: one addresses the needs of incapacitated and isolated people in the community; the other addresses elder abuse and neglect.

As described in Chapter 1, concerns about the growing number of elders and people with disabilities living alone without caregivers led to the passage of Title XX of the Social Security Act in 1975. The act permitted states to use funds, known today as Social Services Block Grants (SSBG) for advocacy and services to adults who, "as a result of physical or mental limitations, are unable to act in their own behalf; are seriously limited in the management of their affairs; are neglected or exploited; or are living in unsafe or hazardous conditions." Although the intent was to prevent or delay institutionalization, early evaluations suggested that APS involvement actually increased clients' likelihood of being admitted to nursing homes (Blenkner, Bloom, Nielson, & Weber, 1974). Although these disappointing results may, at least in part, be accounted for by the inadequate funding most states allocated for APS, interest in APS had already begun to wane by the late 1970s, when elder abuse first came to light.

The emergence of interest in elder abuse in the late 1970s and early 1980s reignited interest in APS. Congressional hearings on elder abuse, which began in the late 1970s, prompted states to enact elder abuse reporting laws (Tatara, 1995). Rather than creating new entities to investigate and provide follow-up, most states assigned their existing APS programs to do the job.

States patterned their elder abuse reporting laws and response systems after those developed for child abuse. The child abuse laws assumed that abused and neglected children were incapable of seeking protection on their own and enlisted the help of teachers, pediatricians, day care workers, and others to report abuse they observe to Child Protective Services (CPS) for investigation and follow-up. Similarly, the elder abuse reporting laws and response system assumed that frail elders could not seek protection on their own and called on professionals and concerned third parties to help.

Abused and neglected elders account for a significant proportion of APS caseloads. The remaining portion includes nonelderly adults with disabilities and self-neglecting adults (Lachs, Berkman, Fulmer, & Horwitz, 1996; Teaster, Dugar, Mendiondo, Abner, & Cecil, 2006).

Because there are no federal regulations for APS, practice varies significantly from state to state and even within states (Mixson, 1995). Typically, however, workers conduct initial assessments that focus on clients' general well-being, including their health, ability to perform daily activities, mental capacity, and living environments. They then work with clients to develop service plans that may include medical care, housing, social services, financial assistance, money management, and support services. The level of service that APS programs provide, and the types of interventions they offer also vary widely. Whereas some offer short-term case management, crisis counseling, safety planning, or assistance obtaining protective orders, most refer clients to other agencies for follow-up services, including counseling, support groups, shelters, legal assistance, or other services they need to stop or treat abuse and prevent its recurrence.

When abuse or neglect are suspected, alleged, or reported, workers investigate, document, and substantiate allegations. In most states, APS workers are required to report to the police if they determine that crimes might have been committed, although some state laws stipulate that workers must get permission to do so from competent clients (Moskowitz, 1998; Roby & Sullivan, 2000). The extent to which APS workers assist in collecting evidence also varies. Some states further require APS workers to notify and interview perpetrators and assess their needs.

Some APS units have taken special steps to enhance their response to abuse victims. These include using specialized assessment instruments, arranging for specialized consultation, and developing protocols for collaborating with other agencies, etc. Some programs have also worked with other agencies in their communities to develop specialized abuse prevention services. These innovations are described in Chapter 6.

Principles Guiding Practice

Adult Protective Services are voluntary, which means that when clients refuse help or fail to cooperate in investigations, workers are obligated to respect their wishes. There are two exceptions:

1. When elders are too impaired to protect themselves, society, acting under the principle of *parens patriae* (the "state as parent"), assumes the right to protect them. Public agencies, for example, can provide involuntary protection such as psychiatric hospitalization for people who pose a threat to themselves or others, or guardianship.
2. Society also has an obligation to protect the public welfare. Acting under "police power," law enforcement officers can intervene to stop harm, the threat of harm, the loss of assets and property, and public nuisances.

A consensus statement developed by the National Adult Protective Services Association (NAPSA) provides guidance to APS workers in how to maximize clients' autonomy (National Adult Protective Services Association, n.d.). The statement cautions workers against imposing their own or society's values on clients and directs them to acknowledge the primacy of clients' interests, as opposed to the interests of society, families, and others when interests compete. Workers are directed to seek informed consent before providing services, respect confidentiality, involve clients in developing service plans, and use family and informal support systems when it is in clients' best interest.

Because many elders referred for APS services have diminished mental capacity, the consensus statement also suggests ways to maximize these clients' ability to exercise choice and autonomy. Workers should assume that clients have capacity unless courts decide otherwise, and when they must exercise authority, they are advised to choose options that are least restrictive and limited in scope or duration.

Benefits and Limitations of the APS Model

APS programs and the abuse reporting systems they work within offer numerous benefits. They provide a critical mechanism and procedures for case identification, investigation, risk assessment, and emergency and short-term interventions in elder abuse cases. Although there has been little research to explore the impact of APS and abuse reporting, that which does exist suggests that the system has been successful in identifying and providing services to elders who might not otherwise have received help. Each year, more and more cases are reported to agencies that can offer assistance (Teaster et al., 2006).

But success has not come without controversy. As described in Chapter 1, APS programs have been the target of frequent criticism from the media, policy makers, other professionals, and clients' families. Some of this criticism undoubtedly stems from lack of understanding about

APS' mandate and workers' commitment to client autonomy. When victims exercise their right to refuse APS investigations and interventions, third-party observers are likely to conclude that the programs are negligent or ineffective. The model's resemblance to the child abuse response system, which is better known to the public, may further create misconceptions and false expectations because CPS workers have much broader powers to prevent abuse, including the authority to remove children from their homes against their wishes when necessary.

As described in Chapter 1, conflicts may also emerge as a result of APS workers' dual role as victim advocates and impartial investigators, which resulted from the merging of APS' federal and state responsibilities. The Texas Community Services Commission pointed out the incompatibility of these two roles in a report to Texas Governor Rick Perry. The commission, which was appointed by the governor in the aftermath of a searing media exposé of the state's APS program, concluded that providing protective services required different skills than those needed to conduct abuse investigations. Furthermore, the commission recommended that the state assess its reporting and follow-up policies and acknowledged the need for additional resources (Mixson, 2005).

APS workers also face uncertainties with respect to such fundamental issues as when involuntary measures are warranted. Although the two exceptions to the voluntary consent rule described earlier may seem straightforward at first blush, determining when clients are incapable of giving (or withholding) consent for services and investigations, and when abuse constitutes criminal conduct, are extremely complicated. There are no universally accepted standards for assessing capacity to consent to APS services, and criminal conduct may not be apparent, particularly during the early stages of abuse investigations.

Other limitations of APS result from the lack of federal guidance, oversight, and coordination, which has resulted in wide variations across the country, and even within states, in how abuse and neglect are defined and who is eligible for services (see Chapter 2). These differences have also made it virtually impossible to develop a national profile of APS or standards for caseload sizes, eligibility for services, and practice in general. There are, for example, enormous differences among states with respect to the number of cases reported, investigated, and substantiated. Jogerst et al. (2003), for example, found that states' rates of reporting ranged from 4.5 to 14.6 per 1,000 elders, investigation rates ranged from 0.5 to 12.1, and substantiation rates ranged from 0.1 to 8.6. This lack of consistency across the country has further delayed efforts to develop a national agenda and priorities. As long as the definitions used to define eligibility for APS services are vague and elastic, it remains impossible to estimate resource needs and ensure that the supply and demand for services will be in sync. Lack of adequate resources has been a constant problem. In a 2001 survey of APS administrators, over 57% cited insufficient resources among their primary problems (Otto & Bell, 2003). As caseloads swell, some APS programs have responded by capping the number of visits workers can make or time spent with them, an approach that runs counter to current understanding of victims' service needs. As described later, current thinking in the field suggests the need for sustained, ongoing contact to overcome the barriers many victims face. As a result of the lack of adequate resources, many APS programs have had to triage cases and serve only those in greatest need.

A final limitation of the APS model is that it does not actually prescribe treatment or therapeutic approaches, but rather, provides a mechanism for receiving and investigating reports and routing clients to others for treatment. As new and promising interventions emerge, it remains to be determined which ones can be integrated into APS practice and which ones are best provided by other agencies. If APS programs assume new roles and responsibilities, they will need to be adequately compensated.

THE DOMESTIC VIOLENCE PREVENTION MODEL

In 1996, I had the pleasure and privilege of interviewing Del Martin for an article on elder domestic violence that appeared in *nexus*, a newsletter for affiliates of the National Committee for the Prevention of Elder Abuse. Ms. Martin authored the seminal book *Battered Lives* (1976, 1981) and coauthored, along with Lenore Walker and Daniel Sonkin, *The Male Batterer: A Treatment Approach*. This is how she described the early days of the domestic violence movement:

> The domestic violence movement has always been a grassroots self-help movement. In the early days, many feminists who had given up on the system got involved. To a great extent, it was women who had left abusive relationships who ran the shelters and led the movement. At one point, we even had an underground railroad to send women who were leaving abusive relationships to other states with other identities. Some women would go from state to state to get away from abusive men. Just leaving a relationship doesn't mean a woman is free. (Nerenberg, 1995)

Other early spokespersons for the domestic violence movement included feminists like Kate Millet (1971) and Susan Brownmiller (1975), who explained domestic violence within the context of gender discrimination and inequalities. According to this "classic" theory of domestic violence, men use physical and sexual violence against their intimate partners to exercise power and control. Overt violence is reinforced by coercion, threats, intimidation, isolation, economic control, and humiliation. Batterers also prevent their victims from seeking outside help. Further, women are vulnerable to violence because of their unequal social, economic, and political status in society, which limit the resources that they have available to them to stop violence (Jewkes, 2002).

Domestic violence theory further holds that public institutions, including the criminal justice system, have supported and legitimized violence against women by treating it as a family matter (Miller, 1994). Historically, "noninterference" was the primary response of police, who were directed not to make arrests unless there were severe injuries or they had personally witnessed the violence (Giacomazzi & Smithey, 2001).

Early studies of domestic violence shed light on how to help victims. Researchers paid particular attention to the "help-seeking process" to understand why, when, and how victims seek help. Because of the formidable economic, cultural, and psychological barriers victims face, they are likely to come forward and retreat many times before they are finally ready to leave abusive relationships. Early studies also suggested that women were at greatest risk when they were planning to leave or immediately after leaving abusers. Others showed that arresting abusers was an effective deterrent to future violence (Sherman & Berk, 1984).

Policy and practice in domestic violence prevention is based on the principle that everyone has the right to live free from violence, and that domestic violence is, therefore, a violation of human rights. The field operates on an "empowerment model," which addresses power imbalances through both *micro* and *macro* interventions. Micro interventions focus on the problems and needs of individuals, whereas macro interventions address those of whole groups and institutions.

A primary goal at the micro level is to help women move past seeing themselves as victims to seeing themselves as "survivors" and taking the lead in protecting themselves. This is accomplished through self-help and legal approaches aimed at overcoming social, economic, and psychological barriers and keeping women safe while they engage in the help-seeking process. Specific interventions and services include the following:

- **Consciousness raising and education** help victims understand domestic violence and facilitate the "help-seeking process."
- **Support groups** provide a forum for members to learn from each other's experiences, recover from trauma, and extend their social support networks.
- **Safety planning** is identifying safe contacts; deciding where to go in emergencies; developing lists of resources such as shelters

and transportation; packing bags with clothes, important documents, and money (and leaving them with trusted individuals); and devising code words to use with family or friends in front of abusers to let them know that they need help. Safety planning is based on the assumption that victims are the experts in knowing when they are in danger and that when they discuss, plan for, and rehearse what to do in advance, they are more likely to take steps when they are in danger.

- **Shelters** provide safe haven from batterers and support.
- **Counseling** helps victims express anger and fear, recognize and appreciate their strengths, set goals, stop blaming themselves, and explore options. In recent years, individual and group therapy has increasingly addressed post-traumatic stress disorder (PTSD).
- **Advocacy** helps women assert their rights and meet their needs with respect to housing, employment, education, public assistance, etc. Court advocacy helps with court-related needs, services, and rights.
- **Civil orders of protection,** which are issued by courts, tell perpetrators to stay away from victims and not to harass or contact them.
- **Financial resources** help victims gain control over their lives. For many women, stopping abuse requires that they achieve financial self-sufficiency.

Macro strategies address the deeply rooted, historic inequalities and discrimination that underlie domestic violence. They include advocating for equal rights, the end to discrimination, and adequate resources so ensure victims' financial independence. They also include advocating for a stronger police response to domestic violence. Criminal justice responses that have been adopted by some states and local jurisdictions include the following:

- **Mandatory arrest policies** require police officers to detain alleged offenders when they have probable cause to believe that the person committed domestic violence.
- **"No-drop" policies** require prosecution of a domestic violence perpetrator, regardless of the victim's wishes, and often force the victim to participate in the process.
- **Evidence-based prosecution.** Recognition that victims are often reluctant to testify against abusers as a result of both explicit and implicit threats or intimidation and other factors has prompted prosecutors to be less reliant on victims' participation in building cases and to rely instead on physical evidence and the testimony of witnesses and experts.

- **Vertical prosecution** is when one attorney handles the same case and victim from beginning to end.
- **Relaxing evidentiary rules regarding "hearsay."** The U.S. Constitution guarantees criminal defendants the right to "be confronted with the witnesses against them," which limits prosecutors' use of "hearsay" testimony in court. Hearsay includes second-hand accounts of out-of-court statements such as 911 calls and criminal complaints or incident reports. The fact that many victims of domestic violence are unwilling to come to court has therefore historically been a barrier to prosecution. Rather than abandon these cases, states began to "relax" the hearsay rule in domestic violence cases, allowing prosecutors greater flexibility to use hearsay evidence and statements. A formidable challenge to this trend came in the form of the Supreme Court's 2004 decision in *Crawford v. Washington,* which is described in Chapter 7.

The domestic violence movement grew rapidly, fueled by grassroots national women's advocacy organizations. These organizations played a prominent role in the passage of the Violence Against Women Act in 1994, which provides for research; education for judges, police, and others; shelters; and enhanced privacy protections for victims. It also criminalized domestic violence, sexual assault, stalking, and violations of protective orders for women. A controversial portion of the act makes gender-motivated crimes a violation of federal civil rights law (42 U.S.C.A. § 13981).

Applying the Domestic Violence Prevention Model to Elder Abuse

In 1992, AARP convened "The Older Battered Woman" symposium, which brought together advocates, researchers, and professionals from the fields of elder abuse and domestic violence prevention to share perspectives and explore the service needs of elderly battered women (AARP, 1993). This groundbreaking event was followed by other important initiatives. In 1996, the Administration on Aging (AoA) of the Department of Health and Human Services funded six model projects to further explore the relationship between elder abuse and domestic violence and approaches to meeting the needs of elderly women. When the Violence Against Women Act (VAWA) was reauthorized in 2001, it included amendments defining elderly women as an underserved population and permitting funds to be used for activities related to elder abuse prevention.

Domestic violence theory and practice was greeted with enthusiasm by many in the field of elder abuse prevention. A first effort to systematically explore the experiences of older women and their needs was undertaken by Carol Seaver, director of one of the nation's first programs designed to serve elderly battered women at the Milwaukee Women's Center (Seaver, 1996). After carefully observing over one hundred elderly battered women, Seaver developed a typology of older battered women. Although there is disagreement today about the categories, experts agree with Seaver's observations that domestic violence continues into old age and that it is often exacerbated by such factors as retirement, the onset of illness and disability, and changing roles. Seaver also observed that many older people enter into abusive relationships in old age.

Seaver and others further observed that older women have needs that are both similar to and different from those of younger women and identified obstacles that older women face in getting help, including illness and disability; financial barriers; caregiving responsibilities; cultural barriers; and physical, communication, and cognitive impairments. They also identified a critical need for outreach to older battered women, particularly those who enter into abusive relationships for the first time late in life. Their work further dispels the common assumption that women who have been in abusive relationships for many years will never leave.

As information and findings emerged from the AoA model projects and other sources, communities began to design new services or adapt existing services to better meet the needs of elderly victims. Services and interventions that have been explored or adapted include support groups, shelters, restraining orders, vertical prosecution and offenders' treatment (Brandl, Hebert, Rozwadowski, & Spangler, 2003; Vinton, 1998; Wolf, 1999).

The response to elder domestic violence varies widely state to state and from community to community. In some states, APS personnel respond to elder domestic violence, whereas in others they do not unless the victim is also vulnerable or dependent as a result of impairment. The extent to which victim service programs serve elderly victims of domestic violence also varies.

Benefits and Limitations of the Domestic Violence Model

Domestic violence theory and practice revolutionized the field of elder abuse prevention. It offered compelling explanations for why some women remain in abusive relationships. It explained how repeated victimization creates fear and hopelessness that entrap and paralyze women, and why they appear to protect or collude with their abusers. The insights into help-seeking that the field introduced forced practitioners in the field of elder abuse prevention to reassess how they worked with victims and taught them promising strategies for overcoming fear, ambivalence, and other impediments to change. It further offered myriad new services and approaches that held promise, not only for victims of elder domestic violence, but for other forms of elder abuse as well. Some programs have attempted to extend definitions, remedies, and services to groups that were not originally protected. For example, a legal services program in San Francisco that pioneered the use of domestic violence restraining orders in elder abuse cases successfully used the orders to restrain adult children of elders; however, the court drew the line when elders sought the orders to restrain nonrelated caregivers.

In recent years, the field of domestic violence has been engulfed in a maelstrom of conflict and controversy. Newer research and appeals by advocacy groups have cast doubt on old assumptions, and led to major revisions in definitions, theory, policy, and practice.

One of the key controversies is the role of gender in domestic violence. The first challenges to the "gender analysis" of domestic violence came from women of color, who argued that, although gender discrimination and inequalities contribute to domestic violence, other forms of oppression and social injustices do so as well. For example, the Sacred Circle National Resource Center, which serves Native women, emphasizes the role that colonization and the disruption of family life resulting from residential schools have played in promoting violence against Native women (Nerenberg, Baldridge, & Benson, 2003). Prominent theorists and advocacy organizations have also acknowledged that racism, classism, heterosexism, ageism, and other forms of discrimination and inequality increase vulnerability to both individual and institutionalized acts of violence (VAWnet). Gay and lesbian antiviolence advocates challenged the role of gender-based power and control disparities altogether by revealing that domestic violence occurs within same-sex couples (Coleman, 1994; Letellier, 1994).

The "men's movement," which originally focused on improving men's rights in regard to marriage and child access, has argued that men are likely to experience domestic violence too, with some prominent researchers suggesting that men are at equal risk as women (Gelles & Loseke, 1993). Some groups have initiated lawsuits claiming unlawful gender discrimination by domestic violence programs that do not serve men, and a 2005 amendment to the Violence Against Women Act specifies that "any grants or other activities for assistance to victims of domestic violence, dating violence, stalking, sexual assault or trafficking in persons shall be construed to cover both male and female victims."

Within our field, there are widespread differences of opinion with respect to the role of gender in elder domestic violence. Several prominent researchers and theorists in Canada and Great Britain have applied a feminist lens to elder domestic violence, emphasizing the significance

of gender inequality in causing and perpetuating elder domestic violence (Aitkin & Griffin, 1996; Hightower, 2002; Neysmith, 1995). So
too, have international forums as described in Chapter 1. However,
groups in the United States have tended to downplay the importance
of women's role in society as a factor contributing to elder domestic violence (and elder abuse in general). Although our colleagues in
domestic violence have come to recognize the shortcomings of focusing
exclusively on gender inequalities and discrimination, thereby ignoring
other salient social forces such as race and class, the tendency by those
in our field to "defeminize" elder domestic violence and ignore social
inequality and injustices altogether is perhaps premature and should be
reconsidered.

In addition to these challenges to theory, questions have also been
raised with respect to practice. For example, although recent studies on
the impact of criminal justice approaches to domestic violence affirm
earlier findings that arrest reduces future violence in some situations,
they suggest that, in others, arrest may actually increase the risk of violence. Specifically, arrest appears to increase the risk among the unemployed (Maxwell, Garner, & Fagan, 2002). Other studies have shown
that arrest reduces violence in the short term, but may increase it in
the long run (Sherman et al., 1991). Other "unintended consequences"
of mandatory arrest policies have been identified. Because the laws do
not typically distinguish between one-time and chronic violence, or
between minor and severe violence, it has resulted in dramatic increases
in the arrest of women as "mutual combatants" despite the fact that
most women are acting in self-defense (Hamberger & Potente, 1994).
Studies of "no-drop" policies suggest that they may actually aggravate
already tumultuous relationships and discourage victims from seeking help. Many of these negative consequences of criminal approaches
to domestic violence appear to be more pronounced for poor women,
women of color, and undocumented immigrant women (Harrison &
Karberg, 2003).

Some feminists have argued that the field of domestic violence has
relied too heavily on criminal justice approaches. Some have claimed,
for example, that these policies limit women's autonomy and that focusing federal domestic violence spending on criminal justice approaches
deflects attention and resources away from women's critical material
needs, which also play a major role in domestic violence (Sullivan &
Bybee, 1999). For example, it has been observed that when advocates
assist battered women access material resources and community services,
women experience less reabuse (Coker, 2004).

Domestic violence theory and practice has offered innumerable
benefits to the field of elder abuse prevention. Many domestic violence

strategies such as shelters, restraining orders, safety planning, and options counseling have become increasingly common. The problems associated with domestic violence laws, however, suggest the need for extreme caution in extending coverage to elderly victims or adapting similar laws for elder abuse. As more cases of elder abuse reach the criminal justice system, we stand to benefit from the insights of our colleagues in the domestic violence movement with respect to the risks, benefits, and unintended consequences of criminal interventions. Hopefully, their guidance will steer us toward promising approaches and away from costly mistakes. As both fields continue to grow and evolve, it will undoubtedly create new opportunities for collaboration and exchange.

THE PUBLIC HEALTH MODEL

In 2001, researchers and service providers from around the country met in Washington, D.C. for the first "Elder Abuse Summit," which was jointly sponsored by the Department of Health and Human Services and the Department of Justice. After two days of discussion, delegates made recommendations and ranked their priorities. Among the most highly-ranked was calling for the Centers for Disease Control and Prevention (CDC) to recognize elder abuse as a "public health and safety issue."

CDC responded favorably by convening a multidisciplinary panel of researchers and representatives from federal agencies, advocacy groups, and medical institutions to discuss elder abuse in 2002 (Ingram, 2003) and, in June, 2007, created an Elder Maltreatment Workgroup. Other groups have also recognized elder abuse as a public health problem, including delegates to the U.N.'s Second World Assembly on Aging in Madrid in 2002. The delegates adopted the "International Plan of Action," which acknowledges elder abuse as a public health problem (United Nations Economic and Social Council, 2002).

What does it mean to address elder abuse as a public health issue, and what is a public health approach?

Public health textbooks invariably refer to the "Broad Street pump incident" as the first public health intervention. In 1854, an outbreak of cholera was sweeping through a district in London. Over 500 people died from the disease within a ten-day period. A physician, John Snow, discovered that what the sick and deceased had in common was that they all lived close to the intersection of Cambridge and Broad Streets, and had gotten water from a single water pump on Broad Street. He convinced city leaders to remove the pump handle, essentially ending the epidemic and launching the field of public health.

What was significant about the doctor's actions was that unlike his colleagues, who were treating individuals with the disease, Snow focused on the "big picture." By figuring out the cause of the disease, who was at risk, and how to curtail its spread, he was treating an entire community. The act of removing the pump handle was also a "preventative" intervention. It prevented people from contracting the disease in the first place.

The history of public health is marked by other important milestones and discoveries. The research methodology associated with public health is epidemiology, which uses statistical analysis to identify patterns, characteristics, and behaviors associated with diseases. People who are found to be statistically more likely to contract disease are considered to be "at risk," and the factors they have in common are called "risk factors." Risk factors may also include characteristics such as gender, race, age, and country of origin that predispose people to problems.

As epidemiology yielded new discoveries about the sources and transmission of diseases, it led to new methods of prevention. It was learned, for example, that some diseases can be prevented through immunization, quarantine, and educating the public about transmission and means of prevention. Diseases linked to behaviors can be prevented by changing those behaviors. For example, the discovery that people who smoke are statistically more likely to contract lung cancer than those who do not led to antismoking campaigns and policy. "Environmental risk factors," such as living in proximity to toxic waste dumps, can be eliminated by removing the hazards or blocking exposure. It was also learned that although some diseases cannot be prevented altogether, their impact can be reduced through early discovery and treatment. Later, the public health approach was applied to injuries and social problems, including domestic violence, as well as to diseases (Dahlberg & Krug, 2002).

The public health approach assumes that government has a responsibility to protect the public. Although many public health interventions are voluntary, government has the authority to use involuntary means and to constrain individuals' autonomy and privacy in the interests of the public's health and safety. Governments can, for example, collect personal health information, compel vaccinations and treatment, and order quarantines. Failure to comply with public health laws constitutes criminal conduct.

Public health practice offers three approaches for preventing diseases and other health and social problems:

- "Primary prevention" focuses on eliminating or reducing risk factors so that problems do not occur in the first place. Vaccinating children, for example, is a public health approach to preventing childhood diseases. It is the preferred approach because it minimizes the human, social, and economic costs.

- "Secondary prevention" identifies and treats people who have risk factors or early signs of problems or diseases.
- "Tertiary prevention" stops problems that are already present, restores people who are affected to their highest function, minimizes the negative effects, prevents disease-related complications, and reduces the chances of recurrence.

Specific strategies and interventions used in the field of public health include:

- **Surveillance** is the ongoing systematic collection, analysis, interpretation, and dissemination of health data. It is used to assess the health status of populations, generate hypotheses about the risk factors associated with diseases, identify public health priorities, and evaluate prevention programs. Many sources of data are used for surveillance, and a first step in public health initiatives is often to identify sources, which may include demographic data, death reports, environmental reports, etc.
- **Screening.** With most diseases and problems, the earlier they are detected, the greater the chances they can be cured or treated successfully. "Universal screening" refers to the practice of screening all patients for certain diseases or problems, in contrast to "targeted screening," which refers to screening members of high-risk groups.
- **Public education** can discourage people from engaging in high-risk behaviors that are associated with diseases such as smoking, driving while intoxicated, or engaging in unprotected sex. Public education can also alert people who at risk for problems and encourage them to get screened. Public health education campaigns are often targeted at high-risk groups.
- **Political or social action.** Some problems can be addressed through laws and policies. For example, Mothers Against Drunk Drivers was highly effective in heightening the penalties for drunk driving.

Applying the Public Health Approach to Elder Abuse

Although interest in the public health model is relatively new, the field of elder abuse prevention has relied on basic public health principles and methodologies for many years. We have, for example, looked at the research on abuse and neglect to identify high-risk groups and used the information to inform practice. Recognizing that elders who live with substance abusing children are at heightened risk has led some practitioners to encourage elderly parents to find other ways to provide support to troubled offspring besides letting them live in their homes. For caregivers, risk reduction strategies include respite care, support groups, counseling, and tools that help them assess and lower their risk of abusing. And the risk of financial abuse can be reduced by education about financial planning that encourages elders to execute advance directives with safeguards against misuse. Furthermore, the American Medical Association has promoted "secondary prevention" by encouraging physicians to universally screen all patients by asking them a set of questions about their experiences with abuse and neglect (AMA, 1992). An important first step to promoting a public health approach to elder abuse was a study commissioned by the National Center on Elder Abuse, which identified over thirty sources of data that currently or could potentially provide data on elder abuse, ranging from APS records to FBI crime statistics (Wood, 2006).

Benefits and Limitations of the Public Health Model

Most people agree that prevention is the preferred approach to addressing diseases and problems because it eliminates pain, suffering, and loss and reduces the need for costly, acute interventions. Public health approaches, however, pose a variety of challenges. In general, preventative approaches to social problems tend to be politically vulnerable. When resources are scarce, policy makers and program planners typically choose to devote them to the most acute problems and situations. This tendency may be accounted for by the fact that documenting the impact of primary prevention or early intervention is complicated. It involves demonstrating that a problem that was likely to occur did not, as a result of preventative measures. Proving why things did not happen is typically much more difficult than proving why they did.

Public health approaches depend on research to identify the risk factors associated with problems. The effectiveness of interventions, therefore, depends on the quality of the research on which the interventions are based. The research on elder abuse is still limited in scope and has yielded inconsistent and often contradictory findings. Naturally, this impedes our ability to make the most effective use of public health methods.

Many of the most successful public health campaigns have been spearheaded by powerful advocacy organizations. Mothers Against Drunk Drivers' successful efforts to raise the penalties for drunk drivers is one notable example. To date, elder abuse has not generated the broad-based and powerful constituency that may be needed to affect social change. Victims and the vulnerable have not advocated for themselves.

THE VICTIM ADVOCACY MODEL

Anyone who watches police dramas on TV can probably recite those famous words: "You have the right to remain silent. Anything you say can and will be used against you in a court of law. You have the right to an attorney." The Miranda warning is one of many rights that the U.S. Constitution grants those who are accused or convicted of crimes, along with the right to be confronted by their accusers, the right to speedy trials, and protections against cruel and unusual punishment.

What comes as a surprise to many is that the Constitution does not offer comparable rights and protections to crime *victims*. Historically, victims have received little support and assistance, and played a very limited role in the criminal cases against their offenders. Because they are considered merely witnesses to the crimes committed against them, victims' views about what should happen to abusers were not considered relevant. In some cases, victims are still not even allowed to be present in the courtrooms where their victimizers are being tried.

It was this lack of attention to victims' needs and concerns that led to the "Victims' Rights Movement," which, like the domestic violence movement, emanated from the social activism of the 1960s and 1970s. Crime victims, including battered women and their advocates, and the families of murder victims, were among the groups responsible for bringing the needs of victims and their families to light.

The federal government also began to recognize during the 1970s that the justice system could not operate effectively without victims' help and began to explore victims' needs (U.S. Department of Justice, Office for Victims of Crime, 1998). In 1972, the National Crime Victimization Survey (CVS) was launched to gain a better understanding of the consequences of crime on victims. Unlike previous crime studies that drew from reported cases, the CVS is based on interviews with a random sample of people who are contacted and asked about their experiences with crime. The survey, therefore, sheds light on unreported, as well as reported, crimes. It found that the actual crime rate was three or four times higher than previously believed (U.S. Department of Justice, Office for Victims of Crime, 1998). In response, the federal government created the Law Enforcement Assistance Administration to increase law enforcement funding, establish victim/witness programs, and sensitize officers to victims' needs.

Other government initiatives followed. In 1982, President Reagan appointed the Task Force on Victims of Crime, which made sixty-eight recommendations for how the public and private sectors could improve the treatment of crime victims. They included a recommendation for a "victims' rights amendment to the U.S. Constitution." Later that year, Congress passed the Federal Victim and Witness Protection Act, which provided for witness protection, restitution, and the fair treatment of victims and witnesses to violent federal crimes.

In 1984, the Victims of Crime Act (VOCA) was passed, establishing the Crime Victims Fund, which is used for victim services and compensation for crime-related losses. The sources of the funds are fines, forfeited bail bonds, and court assessments owed by federally convicted criminal offenders. Most of the funding is believed to come from fines collected from "white-collar" offenders and businesses (Deem, Nerenberg, & Titus, 2007). VOCA also established the Office for Victims of Crime (OVC) within the Department of Justice to implement the Task Force's recommendations and distribute VOCA funds to states. OVC sets regulations for how states can use VOCA funds but still gives them some latitude. VOCA also provides support for demonstration projects, technical assistance, and professional education programs, including training workshops and a national victims academy.

Other important policies that address victims' needs include the Victims' Rights and Restitution Act of 1990, the Violence Against Women Act of 1994, and the Victims' Rights Clarification Act of 1997. Victims' rights have also been addressed at the international level by the United Nations, which, in 1985, adopted a Declaration on Basic Principles of Justice for Victims of Crime and Abuse of Power.

States have also played an important role in advancing victims' rights. A primary focus of advocates has been on amending state constitutions to include victims' rights provisions. So far, over half the states have such provisions. The National Organization of Victim Assistance (NOVA)—an organization of victim service providers, criminal justice professionals, researchers, mental health professionals, and former victims and survivors—has been instrumental in spearheading state initiatives and been at the forefront of a national campaign to enact a federal victims' rights amendment.

Practice in victim advocacy draws from victimology, a branch of criminology that emerged after World War II and studies crime from victims' perspective. It also explores the impact of crime and approaches to helping victims recover. Victimology helps advocates understand victims, their relationships to offenders, and their patterns of seeking help.

The victimology research has followed several threads. Some researchers have attempted to identify risk factors associated with crime including gender, race, economic status, and prior victimization. Because past victimization has been found to be one of the strongest predictors of future victimization, researchers have paid special attention to the victims of multiple or "repeat crimes" like family violence. They have also explored intergenerational patterns, with studies showing that individuals who were abused and neglected as children are much more likely to engage in delinquent behavior during childhood and adolescence, and to be arrested for assault.

Victimology researchers have also explored how victims and witnesses respond to life-threatening events, trauma, or abuse, paying particular attention to post-traumatic stress disorder (PTSD), a response that causes victims to reexperience traumatic events through delusions, hallucinations, flashbacks, and repetitive, intrusive, and distressing recollections or dreams. Victims may also acquire "conditioned responses," which is when certain objects, sounds, or other neutral stimuli trigger intense physiological and emotional responses. To avoid being retraumatized, some victims attempt to avoid thoughts, feelings, activities, or conversations associated with the traumatic events. In some cases, the anxiety may be so great as to impair their ability to carry out routine tasks or activities. The anxiety may also lead to depression or substance abuse. PTSD was added to the Diagnostic and Statistical Manual of Mental Disorders III (a manual used by mental health professionals to diagnose mental illness) in 1980. Although controversial at the time, the diagnosis has gained wide acceptance in the mental health and legal communities since then.

Victimology research has also shed light on the internal processes victims go through in determining if and when to seek help. Although most of the research has focused on violent crime, there has been heightened attention to financial and consumer crimes in recent years.

Victim advocacy is based on the principle that victims have a right to information, a right to be heard in the criminal justice process, and a right to help to make them "whole," or returned to their precrime states. Victims' rights and the specific privileges and services to which victims of crime are entitled have been defined in state constitutions and by national and international organizations. Although they vary, they typically include the following provisions (U.S. Department of Justice, Office of Justice Programs, Office for Victims of Crime, n.d.):

- Protection from intimidation, harassment, and harm
- Notification about the status of their cases, including court proceedings and significant developments
- Information about victims' rights and services
- The right to participate in the criminal justice process by attending hearings and presenting victim impact statements
- The right to confidentiality
- Speedy trials with no unnecessary delays

- Prompt return of property
- Restitution
- Compensation for their losses

Specific interventions and services provided by victim assistance programs, which may be located in public and nonprofit agencies, include the following:

- **Victim/witness protection.** Examples include law enforcement protection from harm or threats; notification when offenders are released, escape, or are moved to less secure facilities; secure waiting areas that separate them from defendants during court proceedings; and "no contact orders."
- **Restitution** is monetary compensation that courts can require offenders to pay victims. Victims often need help documenting their losses and seeking civil or other recourse when offenders do not pay.
- **Victim compensation** covers out-of-pocket expenses related to crimes, including medical bills, counseling, and funeral expenses. Compensation programs are administered by states, usually out of system-based county victim services programs. States establish their own eligibility requirements but must follow federal regulations to receive federal VOCA funds.
- **Victim/witness assistance and advocacy programs.** These programs are usually housed in prosecutors' offices and provide court accompaniment and assistance securing compensation, restitution, and community services. They also provide information about mental health services, support services, resources, and financial assistance and referrals.
- **Mental health services.** A variety of counseling techniques have been explored to help crime victims, with particular attention to PTSD. They include cognitive-behavioral therapy, group therapy, and "exposure therapy" in which victims gradually relive frightening experiences under controlled conditions to help them work through the trauma.
- **Victim impact statements.** These verbal, written, or audio or video-taped accounts of how crimes affect victims are used by courts and probation, parole, and correctional officials in determining sentences and making release decisions. They often provide information that would otherwise not be known. For example, when offenders plead guilty to lesser crimes under plea agreements, judges may not know the full extent to which victims were affected. When victims make statements at parole hearings, which are often long after crimes have been commit-

ted, it helps parole authorities understand the long-term impact of crimes.

Applying the Victim Advocacy Model to Elder Abuse

The field of elder abuse prevention has drawn heavily from the victim advocacy model to understand elderly victims and their needs. Elder abuse researchers have looked to victimology research for guidance in explaining why abuse occurs and who is at risk. Practitioners have looked at counseling, advocacy, and legal interventions to help abuse victims.

Elder abuse researchers have paid particular attention to the "intergenerational transmission of violence" theory, attempting to identify patterns and relationships between different forms of family violence. For example, just as victimology researchers have explored whether mistreated children are more likely to grow up to mistreat their own children or intimate partners, elder abuse researchers have explored whether or not abusive offspring are more likely than others to have been abused by their victims earlier in life. A related theory is learned helplessness, which suggests that people who have been mistreated or witnessed violence during childhood are more likely to be victimized as adults. Although the findings of these studies have been inconclusive, they have revealed promising avenues for further exploration. For example, there is some evidence to support the idea of "pay back": that is, woman or children who have been abused may exact revenge later in life (Kosberg, 1998; Grafstrom, Nordberg, & Winblad, 1992).

Practitioners in the field of elder abuse prevention have also benefited from victim advocates' approaches to counseling and advocacy. For example, counseling programs have increasingly begun to address PTSD. As more cases of elder abuse reach the criminal justice system, elder advocates have learned more about restitution, victim impact statements, compensation, and the need for victim protection.

Despite these developments, elderly victims of crime have not benefited appreciably from services and benefits for crime victims. Victim assistance funds have traditionally been used for domestic violence shelters, rape crisis centers, and child abuse programs. To qualify for victim compensation, victims were originally required to report crimes and cooperate with police and prosecutors in investigations and prosecutions. Because many elderly victims were reluctant to report crimes against family members, and law enforcement officers were reluctant to take reports, few elderly victims met these requirements. In addition, only victims of violent crime qualified for VOCA funds or services, thereby excluding victims of elder financial abuse (Nerenberg, 1999; Deem, 2000; Deem, Nerenberg, & Titus, 2007).

The situation is changing, however, as a result of efforts by OVC to identify and respond to gaps in services. Based on comments solicited from victim assistance and victim compensation program administrators, victim service providers, representatives of national victim organizations, elder services agencies, and others, OVC amended its guidelines in 2001. The revised guidelines encourage states to use VOCA funds to provide services for previously underserved groups, including the elderly. The guidelines also expanded the definition of "elder abuse" to include elderly victims of financial crimes. Although the funds cannot be used to compensate victims for financial or property losses, states can provide mental health services including support groups, respite care, and services for victims with disabilities; credit counseling; and restitution advocacy. The new guidelines further specify that training funds can be used for training APS workers and that emergency shelter can include short-term nursing home shelter for elder abuse victims for whom no other safe, short-term residence is available (OVC, 2002). Because it may be unrealistic to expect vulnerable adults to report to, or fully comply with, law enforcement—as a result of trauma, embarrassment, shame, or cultural factors—the new guidelines permit states to accept reports to APS as an indication of victims' cooperation with law enforcement.

Benefits and Limitations of the Victim Advocacy Model

Despite the growing number of elder abuse cases that are being handled through the criminal justice system, attention to victim advocacy and rights by those in the field of elder abuse prevention has been limited. There have been few attempts to encourage state compensation or assistance programs to focus attention on elderly victims, and few elderly victims are known to benefit from victim compensation and victim assistance programs. This is particularly true in the case of financial crimes. According to the National Center for Victims of Crime, which tracked changes prompted by OVC's revised regulations, victims of violent crime remain the priority in most states. In fact, by 2004, only six states had modified their state laws or procedures to allow VOCA compensation funds to be used for services for financial crime victims (Deem, Nerenberg, & Titus, 2007).

Few elderly victims are believed to receive restitution, which has been attributed to prosecutors' failure to ask for it, judges' failure to order it, and a lack of help for victims to collect what is owed them (Deem, Nerenberg, & Titus, 2007). In addition, restitution orders have limited enforceability because many perpetrators do not have sufficient funds to make repayments. They may also hide assets and income to avoid paying. Many victims lack the resources needed to track down their offender's assets.

However, there are a few programs that have addressed elderly victims' rights and service needs, which are described in Chapter 6. They include prosecutors' offices that have developed specialized senior outreach programs or units aimed at helping elders apply for compensation, access victim services, and pursue restitution.

THE RESTORATIVE JUSTICE MODEL

Restorative justice has been described as a philosophy, a set of practices, a movement, and even a way of life (Raye & Roberts, 2004). Rooted in American Indian and native justice traditions, it addresses crime and abuse as violations of people and relationships, and assumes that certain conflicts, particularly those involving families, can best be resolved by repairing relationships and controlling risk, rather than simply punishing offenders. It is often contrasted with "retributive justice," which focuses on proving guilt and punishing offenders.

The restorative justice movement formally began in 1974 with the first victim-offender reconciliation program (VORP) (Strang & Braithwaite, 2002). It was prompted by a Canadian case in which several young offenders and their victims were offered the opportunity to meet and talk about the crime. The first program in the United States, called victim-offender mediation (VOM), was started shortly afterward and the approach soon spread to Europe. In the 1990s, family group conferencing was introduced by the Maoris in New Zealand and then adopted in Australia. "Peacemaking circles" reemerged from Native American and First Nation tribes.

Restorative justice is based on the premise that victims, their communities, and their offenders all have a stake in repairing the harm caused by crime and ensuring that it is not repeated. All of these "stakeholders" must, therefore, be involved in the justice process. Like victim rights' advocacy, the primary focus of restorative justice is on victims' need for safety, information, validation, restitution, and help to recover and heal. Victims are actively involved, to the extent they want to be, in determining outcomes.

But restorative justice calls for an expanded role for the families of victims and offenders, witnesses, and the broader community. It further acknowledges the importance of these social networks in caring for victims and providing restraints against future crime (Marshall, 1999). Restorative justice also holds that the broader community has obligations and responsibilities for the welfare of members and the social conditions and relationships that promote both crime and community peace. These responsibilities include helping offenders become reintegrated into the community, make amends, and pursue legitimate endeavors. Restorative justice also holds that communities are strengthened if local citizens participate in responding to crime.

Finally, although restorative justice holds offenders accountable, it recognizes that they too may be harmed and in need of healing and reintegration into the community. It offers insight into why they commit crimes and how the criminal justice system influences their likelihood of reoffending. It further addresses offenders' experiences and needs, and provides them with opportunities and encouragement to understand the harm they have caused and take responsibility for it. They are provided with opportunities to express remorse or to ask for forgiveness even though they are not required to do so. Although voluntary participation by offenders is emphasized, those who do not accept their obligations voluntarily are restricted and removed from their communities. This is not, however, intended as vengeance or revenge, and these actions are limited to the minimum necessary to reintegrate them into the community. The goal is that they come out of the "system" better than when they went in.

Restorative justice programs may be carried out with court involvement, under court supervision, or as an alternative to court intervention (Kurki, 1999). When courts are involved, restorative justice interventions may be carried out at different points in the process. For example, programs may be offered to parties as a pretrial diversion, which is an alternative to prosecution that "diverts" certain offenders from traditional criminal justice processing into programs of supervision and services. Other restorative justice programs are offered as a condition of probation or even while offenders are in prison. In the later case, the focus is on offenders' reentry into the community.

There is no single approach to practice, and a variety of techniques are available, which adhere to the following principles:

- All parties involved in crimes should be given opportunities to tell others about their experiences and describe the impact crimes had on them.
- Because all of the parties involved in crime are unique individuals, they are the experts on what matters to them, how to build their relationships, and how best to address the harm. And, because each party has part of the answer, everyone's involvement is needed.
- The emphasis of the process is not on blame, retribution, or finding fault.

- The process is voluntary, and decisions made and actions taken should be determined through consensual decision making.
- The process must be flexible. Because each situation is unique, the parties involved should be allowed to create their own process to the extent possible.

Specific techniques used in restorative justice include the following (Marshall, 1999):

- **Victim-offender mediation,** also referred to as "victim-offender reconciliation" or "victim-offender dialog," is a process in which victims meet offenders in a safe, structured setting and engage in discussions with the help of trained mediators. Victims may tell offenders about the crimes' physical, emotional, and financial impact and ask offenders questions. One common question that haunts many victims is "why me?" Victims are also directly involved in developing restitution plans.
- **Conferences,** which are also referred to as talking circles, accountability circles, and responsibility circles, provide an opportunity for people who are directly and indirectly affected by conflicts to express support for victims and offenders, agree on offenders' responsibilities, consider alternatives, and negotiate outcomes. Participants include victims' and perpetrators' families, friends, supporters, health and social service providers, spiritual advisers, and key community members. Conferencing and circles assume that families know their members' strengths, weaknesses, resources, and who can be counted on. When provided with adequate information, they can, therefore, develop appropriate plans to deal with family problems. Based on traditional tribal justice practices, participants may sit in a circle and pass a "talking piece" (e.g., a feather) from person to person. When participants take the talking piece, others are required to listen. Everyone has the opportunity to describe how the abuse affected him or her and provide input into how the harm should be stopped.

    There are many variations. For example, "sentencing circles" operate within the criminal justice system and are held after guilt has been established. Sentencing circles may operate in different ways: (1) Judges may refer cases to circles to make sentencing recommendations, in which case the agreements made by the circles are then presented back to the judges as recommendations. (2) Alternatively, judges, prosecutors, and defense attorneys may participate in circles, and the agreements reached become the final sentences. In addition, "reentry circles" may

be held to determine conditions of probation and parole. Sometimes separate circles are held for offenders and victims before
they join in shared circles.

- **Community reparative or reparation boards,** which are primarily used for youthful offenders or adult offenders convicted of
nonviolent and minor offenses, are typically composed of trained
citizens who conduct public, face-to-face meetings with offenders
who are ordered by courts to participate. Members of the board
discuss the offenses and their negative consequences, and propose sanctions. The sanctions are then discussed with offenders
until agreements are reached. Finally, the boards develop sanction
agreements and monitor compliance.

Applying the Restorative Justice Model to Elder Abuse

Interest in restorative justice techniques has been growing within the field
of elder abuse prevention, although only a few programs currently exist.
A demonstration project in Washington provided technical assistance to
counties to explore the use of conferencing in resolving conflicts among
caregivers. A similar program has been operating in Waterloo, Ontario.
(Both programs are described in Chapter 5.)

Restorative justice approaches that have been used in related fields
may also hold promise for elder abuse prevention. For example, the
Center for Social Gerontology of Ann Arbor, Michigan has pioneered the
use of mediation as an alternative to guardianship when family caregivers
are in conflict about elders' care. An example of how mediation has been
used to resolve an elder financial abuse case is described in Chapter 5.

Benefits and Limitations of the Restorative Justice Model

Restorative justice is highly controversial. Victim advocates have raised
concerns that the approach pressures victims to forgive offenders before
they are psychologically ready to do so, magnifies their tendency to blame
themselves, and makes them feel like obstructionists if they are unable or
unwilling to overcome anger or distrust. Some suggest that restorative
justice approaches are "soft on crime" and fear that offenders will not
receive their just deserts. Others question the fairness of individualized
responses to crimes rather than punishing criminals equally.

Perhaps the most heated controversy surrounds the use of restorative justice in domestic violence cases. Many domestic violence advocates contend that mediation between victims and abusers is impossible
because of the power imbalances that are deeply rooted in social and
economic injustices and inequalities, and that mediation may even

compound these power and status differences. Some believe that it is dangerous for domestic violence victims. Others argue that expanding the role of families and communities and reducing that of government negates one of the most basic principles of domestic violence advocacy, which is that domestic violence is a public, rather than a private, matter and that "reprivatizing" domestic violence deemphasizes its seriousness (Coker, 2003). Some feminist critics further point out that families and communities often support male control of women and are, therefore, unable or unwilling to support antiviolence measures (Coker, 2003).

Responses to concerns about using restorative justice in domestic violence cases are mixed. Some restorative justice advocates concede that the approach is not appropriate, whereas others point out that victim safety can be assured through careful safety planning (Strang & Braithwaite, 2002). Some even claim that restorative justice approaches are more effective in holding offenders accountable, particularly in certain types of cases like acquaintance sexual assault, which are often dropped or result in acquittal (Daly, Curtis-Fawley, Bouhours, Weber, & Scholl, 2003; Koss, Bachar, & Hopkins, 2003). Because first-time offenders and those who have committed minor crimes typically deny their guilt and are likely to get off with warnings, they never acknowledge or assume responsibility for what they have done.

Although more discussion, research, and practice experience are clearly needed to explore the potential for adapting restorative justice approaches to elder abuse prevention, there are clear incentives for doing so. Many victims want to stop abuse and neglect but also want to see their abusers helped. The approach also holds potential for ensuring greater accountability because criminal prosecution is still relatively rare in elder abuse cases and the likelihood that abusers will be let off is still high. Restorative justice programs can also hold perpetrators accountable for crimes that are less serious than those handled by the criminal justice system or those that cannot be successfully prosecuted.

NEUTRALIZATION THEORY

In the second edition of their seminal book *Elder Abuse and Neglect: Causes, Diagnosis, and Intervention Strategies* (1997), authors Sue Tomita and Mary Joy Quinn describe neutralization theory, which was developed in the 1950s to explain how delinquents justify criminal or antisocial behavior. The material draws from Dr. Tomita's doctoral dissertation in which she made a case for applying the theory to elder abuse and neglect. Although the model has not received widespread attention, it can potentially respond to the frequently asked question "How do abusers justify what they do?" and suggests ways to help offenders redirect their thinking and change their behavior.

According to neutralization theory, many young offenders subscribe to the values of the dominant culture and may even admire honest, law-abiding people (Sykes & Matza, 1957). But these values coexist with deviant values and attitudes that account for their criminal conduct. Unlike people with antisocial personality disorders, who have no regard for the rights of others or the rules of society, these offenders are not indifferent to the disapproval of others. They understand that their offending is wrong, but rationalize their behavior through the following seven "neutralization techniques":

1. Denial of responsibility. Some offenders think of themselves as helpless and predisposed to crime by social forces such as unloving parents, bad neighborhoods, delinquent peers, or poverty.
2. Denial of injury. Some do not see their actions as being wrong because they do not believe that anyone is actually being hurt. Someone who steals a car, for example, may claim that the owner could afford the loss.
3. Denial of the victim. Offenders may see their victims as the wrong-doers or as deserving of punishment or revenge. When they do not know their victims, as is often the case in property crimes, they "deny" them by thinking of them as abstractions, rather than individuals.
4. Condemnation of the condemner. Some offenders believe that those who disapprove of them are hypocrites or deviants, or that they have personal grudges against them. By blaming or attacking their critics, these offenders deflect the focus away from their own wrongdoings.
5. Appealing to higher loyalties. Some offenders subscribe to "higher loyalties," like friendship or the approval of their peers that take precedence over legal constraints.
6. Necessity. Some offenders justify their actions as being necessary.
7. The "metaphor of the ledger." Some feel that if they have good behaviors to their credit, it entitles them to indulge in occasional illegal acts.

Neutralization theory also holds that offenders may "drift" between conventional and criminal behavior, committing crimes when one of two conditions is present, *preparation* and *desperation*. Preparation is coming to the realization that it is possible to commit delinquent acts without getting caught. Desperation is a "mood of fatalism," which causes offenders to feel like they have no control over their surroundings, or are being pushed around or emasculated. Committing delinquent acts gives them back a feeling of control.

Victims may reinforce perpetrators' use of neutralization techniques. They may also believe, for example, that they are at least in part to blame for crimes against them. Perpetrators' denial may further be supported by the social system, as is the case when judges dismiss charges.

Neutralization theory has also been applied to adult criminal conduct. James Coleman (1987) describes how white-collar criminals use neutralization techniques to justify their actions. Most typically, these criminals rationalize their behavior by denying that it caused harm or hurt anyone.

Neutralization theory suggests that offenders can be treated by breaking though their denial. Although the concept of denial is well known to—and frequently used by—counselors and therapists, neutralization theory offers a deeper analysis of the various forms of denial that offenders use. The theory also suggests that different interventions are needed to counter each type of denial. It goes further in suggesting that both victims' and abusers' denial need to be addressed. Because offenders' attitudes and values are deep-rooted and firmly entrenched, neutralization techniques are best employed during the early stages of their criminal careers, or during the "hardening process." Neutralization theory also calls for strengthening the norms against criminal conduct.

Applying Neutralization Theory to Elder Abuse

Tomita and Quinn (1997) provide specific examples of how elder abuse perpetrators use neutralization techniques:

1. Denial of responsibility. Elder abuse perpetrators often claim that their acts were accidents, caused by the stresses of caregiving, or the result of society's failure to provide support or financial assistance. Some contend that illness, alcohol, or drugs "made" them abuse. Victims often support abusers' excuses and blame themselves.
2. Denial of the injury. Both abusers and victims may claim that physical mistreatment is not serious, particularly if it does not require medical attention. Similarly, victims and abusive offspring may rationalize financial exploitation by telling themselves and others that offenders stood to inherit anyway or that their parents can afford to sign away property and other assets.
3. Denial of the victim. Some abusers claim that violence or exploitation was revenge for past abuses committed against them by their victims, or that victims deserved exploitation or

punishment. Abusive caregivers may believe that those they care for are intentionally making their jobs difficult or "faking" disabilities.

4. Condemnation of the condemner. Offenders are using this technique when they claim that APS workers or others are the ones who are abusive or intrusive, or that they are "picking on" the abuser.
5. Appeal to higher loyalties. Abusers who tell victims "If you love me, you won't turn me in," are using this technique.
6. Necessity. Abusers may avoid guilt by convincing themselves that mistreatment was necessary to prevent bigger problems. For example, an abuser may rationalize that withdrawing money from an elder's account is necessary to prevent the elder from squandering it or being exploited by others.
7. The metaphor of the ledger. Victims and their abusers may claim that abusers are good sons, daughters, or caregivers most of the time and are, therefore, entitled to "slip" and commit improper acts once in a while.

Because many acts of elder abuse are committed in private and/or are not discovered, perpetrators are unlikely to be caught or punished. They therefore learn that their actions have no consequences and the risk of being apprehended is low, which reinforces their use of neutralization techniques and makes it likely that they will continue.

Benefits and Limitations of Neutralization Theory

Neutralization theory provides rich insight into the multiple forms of denial perpetrators use and the processes through which they become entrenched. It further suggests how to distinguish abusers who can be helped from those who cannot, and at what points they are most likely to respond favorably to intervention.

The neutralization techniques described above resonate throughout the elder abuse literature although they have not been identified as such. Researchers have, for example, described situations in which previously law-abiding people, when given the opportunity to commit crimes, do so (Wilber and Reynolds, 1996). It might be assumed that when these opportunists are not caught, their behavior is reinforced, which corresponds to the theory's explanation of "preparation."

Unlike the other models described in this chapter, neutralization theory does not offer explicit techniques or services. It has been described as "undeveloped" and difficult to test (Maruna & Copes, 2005). If the model is to be applied to elder abuse, interventions must be developed that respond to each of the neutralization techniques.

THE FAMILY CAREGIVER SUPPORT MODEL

The family caregiver support model is another product of grassroots advocacy. It was championed by Anne Bashkiroff, whose husband's diagnosis of Alzheimer's disease and her quest to find help is described in the poignant *For Sasha, with Love: An Alzheimer's Crusade* (Holland, 1985). It describes Bashkiroff's ordeal of discovering that the disease was progressive and untreatable, and that few services were available. Along with other family caregivers, she launched the San Francisco–based Family Survival Project, which later expanded to become the national Family Caregiver Alliance.

Family caregivers were also instrumental in passing state and federal laws. The earliest public policy initiatives to address caregivers' needs came from the states, which have continued to provide much of the leadership in designing and financing programs for caregivers. States provide funds for services like respite care and allow family members to get paid to provide care under consumer-directed programs. (See Chapter 1.) They have provided tax relief for caregivers and family leave benefits, which allow family members to take unpaid leave to care for ill family members while retaining their health benefits and being guaranteed the same or equal positions when they return to work.

At the federal level, the Family and Medical Leave Act (FMLA), passed in 1993, also provides for family leave, which allows family members who work for employers with fifty or more employees to take up to twelve weeks of unpaid leave a year. The Older American Act's National Family Caregiver Support Program, enacted in 2000, provides additional direct services for caregivers.

The caregiving movement was accompanied by research that focused on the needs of both persons needing care and their caregivers. The early research on caregiving suggested that impaired persons' needs progressed in predictable patterns. When the demands on caregivers reached a critical point, for example, they were likely to experience physical, emotional, and financial consequences, known as "burden." This burden subsequently led to stress, depression, exhaustion, financial problems, and even death. Researchers and advocates proposed that providing services aimed at reducing the demands on caregivers could prevent or reduce burnout.

It soon became apparent that caregiver stress and its impact were more complex than originally believed. The "burden" explanation failed to explain why some caregivers with extremely heavy demands experience little stress, whereas others, with fewer demands, experience high levels. Later studies accounted for these differences by demonstrating the importance of other, subjective factors such as caregivers' negative attitudes about their responsibilities and those they care for (Zarit & Toseland, 1989). Caregivers also found certain behaviors by those they care for, such as incontinence, sleeplessness, wandering, anger, and combativeness, as particularly stressful. The quality of caregivers' and care receivers' relationships prior to the onset of the disability, referred to in the literature as their "premorbid relationship," was also found to be important. When past relationships were good, caregivers experience less stress, even when the demands on them are extremely high. These discoveries suggested new approaches to helping caregivers, such as addressing the tensions and resentments that give rise to stress and helping caregivers find ways to cope.

Practice in the field of family caregiving is based on a "family-systems approach." Family systems theory views families as dynamic and holistic entities that have characteristics in common with all living systems (Hamilton, 1989). They receive "input" from the external environment in the form of support and resources; engage in "core processes," which include communication, interpersonal partnerships, and functions; and respond to the external environment. Dysfunctional behavior results from external stresses, such as economic needs, or internal stresses, such as conflicts between family members, which may be transmitted between generations. It also assumes that all families have strengths, which, when built upon, allow them to change and develop solutions to their problems. This outlook is referred to as a "strengths perspective."

Family systems theory assumes that family systems can be repaired by understanding members' relationships and stresses, identifying strengths and weaknesses, and assessing families' ability to change. Interventions focus on whole families rather that single members. That does not mean that treatment is always directed at whole families, only that practitioners must always be aware of the whole family unit, the clients' ability to function within it, and the likely effect of changes on the family system. Although originally developed for nuclear families, which do not generally include elders, family systems theory was later extended to acknowledge the role of the elder generation on nuclear families.

In keeping with the family systems approach, the goal of practice in the field of caregiving is to identify and resolve stresses within families and build upon their strengths to help them remain intact and function better. It assumes that families, rather than individuals, are the clients. Specific interventions include the following (Gallagher-Thompson, 1994):

- **Caregiver education and training programs** focus on patients' diagnoses and their implications, how to plan for future care needs, and community services.
- **Long-term-care planning and case management** address the needs of both impaired persons and their families, helping them explore care options, arrange support services, respond to crises, and adjust to daily routines.

- **Caregiver support groups** provide emotional support, instruction, and guidance in how to meet care receivers' needs and handle difficult behaviors. They may further address the tensions and resentments that give rise to stress.
- **Social support,** which includes informal recreational and social activities, reduces the loneliness or isolation that many caregivers experience.
- **Respite programs** relieve caregivers for a few hours or for extended periods. Elders may come to agencies, day centers, or long-term care facilities to give their caregivers a break; or, alternatively, attendants, professionals, or volunteers may come to their homes.
- **Support services**—which include daily money management, home delivered meals, attendant care, transportation, friendly visitors, and telephone reassurance—decrease elders' reliance on their caregivers while also reducing pressures on caregivers.
- **Counseling** helps families solve problems and develop coping skills.
- **Legal and financial planning** helps families with estate planning, advance directives, guardianships, and other matters.
- **Financial incentives and compensation** include direct payments to families, through cash grants or vouchers, to purchase services. Tax incentives for caregiving include deductions and credits.

Applying the Family Caregiver Support Model to Elder Abuse

The early research on elder abuse closely paralleled the research on caregiving. Early studies on elder abuse were based on many of the same premises, including the assumption that the more care elders required from their caregivers, the more stress their caregivers experienced. Elder abuse researchers took the premise a step further, postulating that when caregivers' stress levels reached a critical point, they resorted to abuse or neglect.

But just as caregiving researchers came to recognize that caregivers' attitudes about caregiving and their relationships with those they cared for were equally, if not more, important than the amount of care they provided in causing stress, so too did elder abuse researchers come to recognize the importance of these factors. For example, some elder abuser researchers also found that abuse was closely linked to the quality of premorbid relationships and to disturbing behaviors by care receivers, including aggression, combativeness, and violence (Anetzberger, 1987;

Compton, Flanagan, & Gregg, 1997; Heath et al., 2005; Pillemer & Suitor, 1992). It was also discovered that abusive caregivers were more likely than nonabusive ones to feel that they were not receiving adequate help or support from their families or the social service system (Anetzberger, 1987; Compton et al., 1997).

Other important discoveries regarding abuse by caregivers included the observation that abuse is often two-directional and may be triggered by aggressive care receivers; that certain stresses affect both caregivers and patients and may trigger aggression in either or both; and that depression is predictive of abuse in either direction (Hansberry, Chen, & Gorbien, 2005; Paveza et al., 1992; Quayhagen et al., 1997). These discoveries about the interactive nature of abuse in caregiving relationships have led some researchers to look at pairs, or "dyads," of caregivers and care receivers, and to think of "families at risk." Another important finding was that as many as 50% of caregivers for people with dementia are fearful that they will abuse those they care for even though only a small percentage actually do (Pillemer & Suitor, 1992).

Despite the likely relationships between caregiver stress and elder abuse, there have only been a few service programs designed to help caregivers lower their risk of abusing. They include self-assessment tools to help caregivers assess their risk and caregiver support groups that reduce members' isolation, help them explore negative feelings, and explore ways to change abusive behaviors (Podnieks & Baillie, 1995; Reis & Nahmiash, 1995; Scogin et al., 1989). Conferencing (as explained under the Restorative Justice model) has also been explored as way to help caregiving families resolve conflicts. These programs and resources are described in Chapter 5.

Benefits and Limitations of the Caregiving Model

Addressing elder abuse as a "caregiver issue" has been the topic of considerable controversy in the field of elder abuse prevention. Some believe that given the relational dynamics between elders and their caregivers and the risk of abuse they pose, the field must address abusers' needs for support services (Baron & Welty, 1996; Bergeron & Gray, 2003). Others, however, believe that too much emphasis has been placed on caregivers' needs already and that it has diverted attention away from more promising approaches. For example, some suggest that viewing abuse as a "caregiving issue" discourages practitioners from assessing for domestic violence, thereby leading to inappropriate interventions that can place victims, particularly battered women, in danger (Brandl & Raymond, 1997). A related concern is that caregiver stress will be used as an inappropriate defense or excuse for abuse, thereby letting abusers off the hook.

Clearly, caregiver stress is not the only explanation for elder abuse, and abusive caregivers need to be held accountable. However, failure to acknowledge and address the very real demands that many caregivers face and the interactive nature of abuse between caregivers and those they care for, would be equally misguided. These needs will clearly become more acute in light of the Olmstead decision, described in Chapter 1, which has already resulted in increasingly frail individuals living in the community. This in turn is placing greater demands on family caregivers. As Lynn Friss Feinberg, deputy director of the National Center on Caregiving at the Family Caregiver Alliance states, "Caregivers are doing things today that would make nursing students pale" (Feinberg, 2006).

Nowhere are the demands on caregivers more intense than in communities of color. The shortage of family caregivers, and the overwhelming demands that caregivers face, have been common themes in the literature on abuse against Native American, African American, and Hispanic elders (see Chapter 4).

Concerns about excusing abusive caregivers' behavior are clearly understandable. But failing to address caregivers' needs and overemphasizing culpability may keep caregiving families from getting the services they need to reduce their risk of abusing. If caregivers feel that they will be unfairly treated, it is unlikely that they will be willing to disclose negative feelings about those they care for, their fears about committing abuse, or problems they are having in managing care receivers' aggressive or violent behavior. Similarly, professionals who work with caregivers will be unlikely to report if they feel that their clients will be treated unfairly.

These problems can be avoided by recognizing that there is no single approach to treating abuse and neglect by caregivers. Determining when abusive caregivers should be provided with support services and when they should be punished or relieved of their responsibility is best determined on a case-by-case basis. Professionals in the fields of dementia care, as well as those in the fields of APS and law enforcement, need to come together to help each other better understand the dynamics in these cases, the needs of caregivers, and what constitutes unacceptable behavior.

Cross-disciplinary education is also needed. Those working with caregivers need instruction in elder abuse prevention, including how to assess and handle high-risk situations such as poor past relationships, previous histories of family violence, and caregivers' fears of becoming violent. They further need direction in how and when to report, the benefits of reporting, how to develop safety plans, and how to handle dangerous situations such as when elders with dementias have weapons. Law enforcement, prosecutors, judges, and others need training to help them evaluate "caregiver stress defenses" and help them differentiate legitimate from bogus explanations.

Caregiver support programs, APS, domestic violence programs, and criminal justice approaches need not be in conflict when it comes to handling abuse by caregivers. Working in tandem with caregiving programs, the criminal justice system can provide powerful incentives and leverage for abusive caregivers to get help and treatment. An exploratory program in New York, for example, which is patterned after programs for domestic violence offenders, provides education to abusive caregivers, most of whom are court-ordered into the program. The program is described in Chapter 5.

THE FAMILY PRESERVATION MODEL

In an intriguing article entitled "Family Preservation: An Unidentified Approach in Elder Abuse Protection," Rene Bergeron, associate professor of social work at the University of New Hampshire, explains how a model that is rarely discussed in relation to elder abuse prevention, has, in fact, played a significant role in shaping practice (Bergeron, 2001).

The family preservation model, which was developed in the 1980s, assumes that the most effective way to prevent child abuse and neglect is to work with families rather than removing children from their homes or separating them (Kelly & Blythe, 2000). Bergeron suggests that APS workers, many of whom worked in child protective services before coming to APS (Jogerst, Daly, & Ingram, 2001) have integrated key components of the model into their work with abused and neglected adults.

The family preservation model, like the caregiver support model described in the previous section, is based on family systems theory. Its goal is to help families remain intact. This is accomplished by identifying and addressing stresses within families and building upon strengths. Families, rather than individuals, are the clients.

Family preservation practice also draws from and shares goals with family therapy and counseling. Practitioners help families understand their dynamics and changes. They discuss problems, negotiate responsibilities, and delegate tasks. Instruments and techniques like family trees or *genograms* (charts of social and familial relationships) are sometimes used to graphically depict and explain family strengths and weaknesses, identify conflicts, and set goals. Assessment tools have also been developed to help clinicians recognize family strains and note changes over time within family systems.

Working in the family preservation mode, practitioners develop service plans to reduce stress, resolve conflict, support families, and monitor risk. In doing so, they build on family strengths and consider how changes will affect family systems.

Because family preservation sees each family as unique, interventions vary from family to family. Practice in the field can, however, be characterized by several criteria, which Bergeron (2001) identified:

- Small caseloads
- Several clients within a family
- Providing intensive, short-term treatment to families within their homes to develop a complete picture of the abusive situation, build trust, and avoid contributing to the families' stress
- A "strengths perspective," which assumes that clients and their families have the ability to change and are important partners in developing solutions
- The use of informal and formal services to reduce family stress, increase caregivers' skills, and manage conflict; includes providing or connecting families with appropriate community services
- Ongoing monitoring of the abusive home to ensure abuse is not recurring
- Education in caregiving and conflict management skills
- Flexible and creative practice approaches that use experimentation and improvisation

Applying the Family Preservation Model to Elder Abuse

Although, as Bergeron points out, there has been little discussion about the family preservation model, its influence is apparent in elder abuse research and practice. Bergeron, in fact, suggests that many states' elder abuse laws dictate a family approach by mandating APS to notify perpetrators about investigations, interview them about victim's needs, assess their needs, and involve them in the development of solutions, which may involve providing them with services.

Family preservation interpretations and techniques are also evidenced in APS workers' perceptions about their work. Bergeron interviewed fifteen APS workers in New Hampshire, all of whom described themselves as "family workers," whose role was to help both victims and perpetrators. Almost half further viewed themselves as advocates for both perpetrators and victims; advocacy for perpetrators included reducing their dependency on victims. Other family preservation practice techniques they use include conducting multiple and intensive visits, assessing and monitoring risk, linking families with informal and formal services, building family support networks, and ongoing case monitoring.

Occasionally, the use of family preservation and family systems approaches are more apparent. An elder abuse multidisciplinary team in one community, for example, uses genograms to help team members understand familial relationships between individuals in the cases being discussed (Teaster & Nerenberg, 2003). In addition, some elder abuse practitioners have endorsed the use of short-term family therapy with abusive or high-risk families (McDaniel, Lusterman, & Philpot, 2001; Williams-Burgess & Kimball, 1992).

Researchers in elder abuse have also looked to the research on families to identify and understand the factors and dynamics that contribute to or trigger abuse, including intergenerational patterns of family violence, caregiver stress, and dependency. Hamilton (1989), for example, uses a family systems interpretation to explain how the onset of disability may disrupt members' previous ways of relating to each other and introduced REAH, an assessment tool that was created to avert elder abuse. The tool identifies family strain, noting changes over time within family systems, evaluating risk, and developing appropriate interventions and referrals (Hamilton, 1989). Drayton-Hargrove (2000) also offers guidelines for assessing families at risk for elder abuse using a family systems approach.

Benefits and Limitations of the Family Preservation Model

Adapting the family preservation model and family systems theory to elder abuse prevention makes sense in light of the fact that most elder abuse is committed by family members. In addition, many elderly victims prefer solutions that keep their families intact, with some even valuing their families' welfare above their own safety. Many elderly victims want to help troubled abusive offspring and feel responsible for them, particularly those abusers who have developmental disabilities or mental illnesses, or who have substance abuse or financial problems. The model's goal of keeping families together by resolving conflicts and mediating solutions is therefore compatible with the elder abuse field's commitment to self-determination.

Other potential benefits of the model for elder abuse prevention include its flexibility. Because victims are often reluctant to accept help, APS workers may need to remain engaged with and connected to families over time and even provide services that are not directly related to the abuse. The family preservation model provides this flexibility. It acknowledges the important role that families play in caregiving and long term care, and recognizes that many abused elders are dependent on perpetrators for services and to remain living in the community. This is particularly true in rural areas where services and housing are particularly scarce. Helping families resolve conflicts can reduce the need for outside supports.

If the family preservation model gains acceptance in elder abuse prevention, it may arouse controversy similar to that raised by the family caregiver model. As described earlier, many domestic violence advocates contend that interventions aimed at resolving conflict between partners in violent relationships are not recommended, at least until batterers have accepted responsibility for their violence. However, the fact that such prominent domestic violence organizations as the Family Violence Prevention Fund have acknowledged the important role that family preservation practitioners can play in identifying domestic violence and ensuring the safety of victims and witnesses, including children, bodes well for resolving these differences (Schechter & Ganley, 1995). Clearly more discussion and research is needed to determine when the approach is appropriate.

Another potential obstacle to employing the family preservation model in elder abuse prevention is that it is relatively expensive. The approach requires intensive short-term interventions with multiple clients, followed by long term monitoring, which many states cannot currently afford. Although the approach has been credited with reducing the need for other more costly services such as alternative housing, the extent to which these savings can be realized remains to be demonstrated. There is also no empirical evidence demonstrating the family preservation model's effectiveness in keeping elderly parents and other family members together. As Olinger (1991) points out, however, identifying the current role and benefits of the family preservation approach may prompt local, state, and federal policy makers to reexamine caseload size, educational requirements, supervision, and program funding for elder abuse prevention workers.

CONCLUSION

The models described in this chapter provide a rich array of options for crafting our own comprehensive elder abuse prevention service delivery model. They provide strategies to keep victims safe and help them heal, hold perpetrators' accountable for their acts and steer them away from counterproductive paths, support families, and even strengthen whole communities. They can help us respond to new, emergent needs.

In the past, some in our field have championed certain models and rejected others. This notion that one model is better than, or trumps, others is counterproductive. It is unrealistic to assume that any single approach can meet the needs of each and every situation as well as the needs of victims, abusers, families, and society. Adopting domestic violence approaches does not preclude support to caregivers, and empowering victims does not require us to abandon perpetrators. Although advocating for individual victims is the preferred approach in some cases, working with families may be appropriate for others.

Despite the advantages of borrowing approaches designed for other populations, it can pose risks. For example, patterning the elder abuse reporting laws and response systems on those designed to protect children originally saved time and effort but also led to ongoing misunderstanding and required countless revisions and adaptations. In our enthusiasm for domestic violence approaches, we need to guard against overextending the model and exposing our clients to unintended consequences. In taking a cafeteria approach to models, we need to carefully choose those aspects of models that serve our needs, proactively explore their pitfalls as well as their benefits, and choose carefully.

The models that are presented here have different and conflicting goals. In presenting them, it is hoped that readers will achieve a clearer understanding of the rationales, ideologies, constituencies, and histories that drove their development. We can also learn from the struggles, successes, and failures of those who advanced them. And finally, it is my hope that in achieving a clearer understanding of those networks that inspired and nourished ours, it will suggest opportunities for future collaboration. We have much to gain by doing so. Some opportunities for collaboration are explored in Chapter 10.

CHAPTER FOUR

Factors Influencing
Intervention Needs

INTRODUCTION

As the last chapter underscores, the field of elder abuse prevention has an abundance of promising models and approaches to draw from in helping victims and holding perpetrators accountable. How then, do we decide what approaches are the most appropriate and effective?

Clearly, given our field's commitment to client autonomy, in most cases, the foremost consideration is what victims want. The primary goal is to help them explore and exercise their options. Clients' wishes, however, have to be considered in light of their abilities, limitations, and resources. In some cases, victims' wishes and needs also have to be weighed against other societal goals, such as keeping the public safe and protecting those who are incapable of protecting themselves.

Perpetrators also need to be considered. The level of risk they pose; their reasons and motives for abusing; their relationships to their victims; and their willingness and ability to stop abusing, make amends, and participate in treatment also need to be taken into account. Other critical considerations in developing service plans include the severity of the abuse and the urgency of victims' need for help. Service providers are also guided by professional ethics and practice principles. And finally, the cultural context in which abuse occurs is crucial to intervening effectively.

This chapter summarizes all of these factors, setting the stage for Chapter 5, which describes specific services and interventions.

VICTIM CONSIDERATIONS IN DEVELOPING SERVICE PLANS

Victims of abuse and neglect vary widely. Some are frail and depend on others for care, whereas others are healthy and independent. Some reside in nursing homes, some live alone, and others live with spouses or adult children. Some are capable of making decisions for themselves, whereas others need surrogates to act on their behalf. Victims also differ with respect to gender, culture, age, and financial resources.

Among the most significant considerations in service planning are victims' cognitive abilities, their ability to make decisions about their care, their willingness to accept services, the factors that place them at risk, and their resources.

Victims' Mental Capacity and Ability to Consent

Victims' mental capacity is a critical consideration in service planning. It determines the extent to which victims can participate in planning for their own care and the interventions that are needed and available to them.

The term *capacity* warrants explanation. In the past, people who were diagnosed with dementias or began to show signs of confusion or forgetfulness were likely to be labeled *incompetent*, a term that is imprecise and highly stigmatizing. Current thinking acknowledges that cognition is a cluster of mental abilities that we use in our everyday lives, and that different skills are needed for different mental tasks. For example, balancing a checkbook requires different skills than remembering to turn off the stove. Dementias, accidents, or normal decline lead to deficits in certain cognitive abilities and, consequently, prevent people from performing certain tasks while remaining capable of performing others. For that reason, when people are diagnosed with dementias or begin to show signs of having problems, their abilities and disabilities need to be carefully assessed so that they are only helped with those tasks and responsibilities they are incapable of carrying out. The term *incapable* begs the question "incapable of what?"

Intervening in elder abuse cases often requires evaluating clients' decision-making capacity, which is one aspect of overall capacity. Decision-making capacity refers to people's ability to make and communicate decisions, understand the consequences of their actions, and act in their own self-interest, and it too, is task-specific. Determining whether someone has decision-making capacity requires looking at the decision in question and whether the person has the mental skills that are needed to understand the decision and its consequences.

Professionals are generally in agreement about how to evaluate decision-making capacity for certain decisions but not others. For example,

Table 4.1   Criteria for Assessing Capacity for Specific Tasks

Decision or Action	Criteria
Capacity to contract	The person must be able to understand the nature and consequences of the transaction.
Capacity to give gifts (donative)	The person must have "an intelligent perception and understanding of the dispositions made of property and the person and objects one desires shall be the recipients of one's bounty."
Capacity to create or revoke a power of attorney	Traditionally based on the capacity to contract although some courts have held that the standard is similar to that for making a will.
Capacity to make medical decisions or execute advance health care directives	The patient must have the ability to • Understand the medical problem • Understand the proposed treatment • Understand alternatives to the proposed treatment • Understand and appreciate the foreseeable benefits and risks of the treatment and of postponing or refusing it • Communicate decisions

because people have been contesting wills for centuries, there is general agreement among lawyers about "testamentary capacity," which is the capacity needed to execute wills: people must understand what a will is, have a basic plan for distributing their assets to heirs, know the nature and extent of their assets, and be able to identify or recognize potential heirs and beneficiaries. There is less agreement, however, about how to evaluate other decisions that are commonly questioned in elder abuse cases. These include the capacity to get married, give gifts, consent to sexual relations, select and supervise home care workers, and accept or refuse services. Table 4.1 gives examples of criteria that are commonly used in assessing decision-making capacity for decisions.

Capacity to Consent

One form of decision-making capacity that workers often need to assess is clients' ability to give *consent*, which is agreeing to actions, transactions, or services proposed by others. Capacity to consent requires that the person understands the act or transaction, is acting freely and voluntarily, and is not under the influence of threats, force, or duress. In the case of informed consent for financial decision making, for example, the person making a transaction must be provided with information and have the mental capacity to understand and appreciate it.

Furthermore, they must be acting voluntarily and be free from coercion (Naimark, 2001).

Consenting to Services

Determining if clients are capable of consenting to services is among the first determinations that service providers often make in care planning. Consent requires that would-be clients have information about the services being offered, understand them, and act freely.

Professionals have developed the following four categories to characterize clients' ability and willingness to accept help and the role of helping professionals in working with each type:

- Capable and consenting. When capable clients consent to help, their workers' role is to provide them with information and help them evaluate their options. Workers must be willing to accept clients' choices, even if they disagree with them.
- Capable and nonconsenting. When capable clients refuse help, those working with them have to respect their wishes.
- Incapable and consenting. Some clients who are deemed incapable of making decisions nonetheless consent to services. Although providing services to them raises ethical questions (workers may be accused of only questioning the capacity of clients who disagree with them), most agencies respect these clients' wishes to the extent that they seem reasonable and appropriate.
- Incapable and nonconsenting. When clients who lack capacity refuse needed services, and the potential consequences of failure to act are serious, involuntary interventions such as protective custody or guardianship may be needed.

Although these categories may seem straightforward, in reality, deciding when clients are capable and consenting can be extremely difficult. There is no universal standard for defining capacity to consent to services, and few agencies have clear guidelines. Clients' capacity may fluctuate over time and is affected by poor nutrition, depression, interactions between medications, and even the time of day (some people are more alert at certain times of day than at others).

In recent years, practitioners have come to understand that victims refuse help because of fear, shame, despair, or distrust. As described in Chapter 1, we now have a better grasp of how perpetrators exercise power, control, and undue influence over victims. Because victims' initial reluctance to accept help can often be overcome by addressing these factors in the early stages of interventions, seasoned workers may avoid directly asking prospective clients for "consent," and focus instead on establishing rapport and developing trust.

As APS expert Paula Mixson (2005) points out,

> The easy decisions are at either end of the (capacity) spectrum, but more often case situations fall into the middle ground. In this territory, when the danger is not immediate and the client has questionable capacity, experts such as ethicist Harry Moody argue that the proper course is "negotiated consent," the use of persuasion, advocacy, and empowerment to induce change (Moody, 1988). Negotiated consent requires spending time with clients, getting to know them, letting them get to know you, and building up trust and rapport so they will be willing to make the needed changes.

Clients who refuse protective services may sometimes be willing to accept support services like home-delivered meals, visitors from volunteer or church programs, telephone reassurance, or social clubs. All of these services can be helpful in reducing isolation, enhancing workers' credibility, and making sure that elders have someone to talk to if they change their minds about services or if the abuse gets worse.

When clients' capacity to accept or refuse services is unclear, workers typically weigh the potential consequences of not intervening against those of doing so. Generally, it is best to err on the side of intervention, particularly when the interventions under consideration are health or social services, which do not pose a serious risk to clients' freedom or autonomy. When the potential consequences are serious (e.g., the risk of abuse is high or involuntary interventions are being considered), more comprehensive assessments, such as "dementia workups" or neuropsychological tests are considered (see Chapter 5).

Decisions to intervene or not to intervene can have serious repercussions in elder abuse and neglect cases. Failure to intervene may result in injury, decline, financial loss, or even death. Workers and agencies may be accused of negligence or incompetence. On the other hand, when workers initiate involuntary protective interventions, they may be accused of paternalism or authoritarianism. In controversial cases, workers may be called upon to defend their actions to other professionals, victims' families, courts, professional boards, or the media.

Factors to consider in evaluating clients' capacity to refuse or to consent to services:

- When capable clients refuse help, what are the potential reasons? Can their fears, distrust, or depression be overcome?
- Are clients who refuse protective services willing to accept support services or to have workers check in on them from time to time?

- When elders show signs of diminished capacity, what are the potential causes? Is it permanent or treatable? Can capacity be enhanced?
- What are the risks to nonconsenting clients? Do they warrant involuntary interventions? What involuntary interventions are available?

Victim Risk Factors

The factors that place elders at risk for abuse also dictate their service needs. Table 4.2 provides examples of victims' risk factors for elder abuse.[1]

Victims' Resources and Support Systems

Victims' family networks, friends, churches, community groups, and civic organizations can play an important role in preventing abuse and helping them recover. These informal networks can provide emotional support and encouragement to victims, help them seek safety, provide relief to caregivers, and alert others to victims' and caregivers' needs. Sometimes, members of clients' informal support networks distance themselves or withdraw support when professionals get involved believing that their help is longer needed or that their involvement will be viewed as interference. Others may withdraw out of distrust. It may therefore be advisable for services providers to develop relationships with these entities (as long as clients agree to it) and encourage them to remain involved. It should be noted though that informal support networks are sometimes the source of distress or confusion.

Victims' financial resources and their willingness (or the willingness of their families) to purchase services also determine what options are available. Clients who can afford to pay for services are likely to have more options available to them in light of the many new, for-profit services that have emerged in recent years. These include professional fiduciaries, geriatric care managers, elder law attorneys, and money managers.

Although for-profit providers may be able to respond more quickly and exercise greater flexibility, those working with abused elders should not assume that for-profit services are preferable to those offered by public or nonprofit agencies. Public and private nonprofit agencies may have resources and authority that for-profit businesses lack. For example, some communities have multidisciplinary teams that are only available to professionals from the nonprofit sector, giving members a broader and more diverse range of experts to consult with. When referring clients to for-profit health and social services, workers must be extremely careful to make referrals to reputable organizations and to be fair and impartial. Many public agencies have protocols for making referrals to private practitioners such as elder law attorneys and financial managers.

Table 4.2   Victims' Risk Factors and Associated Characteristics

Victims' Characteristics with Respect to	Associated Risk Factors
Health and functional ability	• Elders in poor health and who have functional limitations are at heightened risk (Beach et al., 2005; Fisher & Regan, 2006; Lachs & Pillemer, 1995). • Because neglect involves elders who depend on others for care, neglect victims tend to be in poor health and have functional limitations. • Certain types of abuse presume cognitive impairment. For example, inducing someone who lacks decision-making capacity to surrender property is a form of financial abuse.
Dementia and mental health problems	• Some studies show that victims are more likely than nonvictims to have dementias. Some suggest that it is violent or disruptive dementia-related behavior that increases risk (National Research Council, 2003; Pillemer & Suitor, 1992). • Victims are likely to experience mental health problems, including depression, low self-esteem, and substance abuse (Dyer, Pavlik, Murphy, & Hyman, 2000; Fisher & Regan, 2006).
Isolation and lack of social support	• Victims are likely to be socially isolated (Brozowski & Hall, 2004; Compton et al., 1997; Lachs et al., 1994).
Gender	• Household surveys suggest that men are more likely than women to be abused. This may be explained in part by the fact that men are more likely to live with others, which increases their risk (Pillemer & Finkelhor, 1988; Podnieks, 1992). • Most reported cases of abuse and neglect, however, involve female victims. This is true for all forms of elder abuse except abandonment (National Center on Elder Abuse, 1998). • The ratio of women to men varies by the type of abuse. Women are only slightly more likely to experience neglect but much more likely to experience domestic violence and sexual assault (National Center on Elder Abuse, 1998). • The preponderance of reports involving women may be due to the fact that there are more elderly women and that women experience greater physical and emotional harm (Pillemer & Finkelhor, 1988).

Table 4.2   (*Continued*)

Victims' Characteristics with Respect to	Associated Risk Factors
Age	• The risk of abuse increases with age. Elders eighty years old and older are two to three times more likely than other elders to be the victims of all categories of abuse (National Center on Elder Abuse, 1998).
Ethnicity	• Caucasians have the highest percentage of abuse; they constitute eight out of ten reported cases for most types of maltreatment (National Center on Elder Abuse, 1998).
	• Elderly African Americans appear to be at heightened risk (Lachs et al., 1994; NCEA, 1998).
Living arrangement	• Victims are likely to live with others (Lachs & Pillemer, 2004; National Research Council, 2003; Pillemer & Finkelhor, 1988; Paveza et al., 1992).
	• Residents of skilled nursing facilities are among society's most frail members. The following residents are believed to be at particularly high risk:
	• Those who lack family, friends, or advocates (Meddaugh, 1993; Menio, 1996)
	• Those with cognitive and physical limitations (Burgess, Dowdell, & Prentky, 2000)
	• Those on public assistance (facilities may receive lower reimbursement levels)
	• Those who are physically or verbally aggressive (Pillemer & Moore, 1989)
Suffered recent losses	• The loss of a spouse or other family member may increase elders' need for care, which, when not responded to, results in neglect.
	• Recently widowed elders who are managing finances for the first time are believed to be at heightened risk for financial abuse (Blunt, 1993).
	• Some financial predators target recent widows and persons who are declining physically (Deem, Nerenberg, & Titus, 2007).
Lack of resources	• Elders who are unable to purchase services are more dependent on family members and others for help, thereby raising their risk of neglect and self-neglect (Duke, 1991).

Factors to consider in assessing clients' resources include the following:

- Does the elder have family, neighbors, friends, or spiritual advisers who can help or monitor the situation?
- What public and private services are available to clients? What are their benefits and limitations?
- If elders are able and willing to purchase services, what are the benefits and risks of doing so?

PERPETRATOR CONSIDERATIONS

Perpetrators' characteristics, their relationships to their victims, the ongoing risk they pose, their reasons for abusing, and their willingness and ability to stop abusing and make amends all need to be considered in determining what services and interventions are available and appropriate to stop abuse.

Perpetrators of elder abuse range from spouses to paid caregivers to corporate entities (e.g., when abuse occurs in long-term care facilities). Some have financial motives, whereas others abuse out of frustration or anger. Some have malevolent motives, whereas others, including those with mental illnesses or dementias, are driven by impulses beyond their control. Some feel remorse for what they have done and want to make amends, whereas others are continually on the lookout for new victims.

The terminology used to describe perpetrators' relationships with their victims can be confusing. The term *caregiver* refers to paid employees as well as family members and friends who provide care informally. Informal caregivers may help out voluntarily or have a "duty of care" as defined by law. However, as described in Chapter 2, the extent to which family members are legally responsible to provide care and the type of care required has not been clearly established and varies by state. And, as described in Chapter 1, family caregivers are increasingly receiving payment through public entitlement programs.

Paid caregivers may work for licensed agencies that screen, schedule, supervise, and pay them. This is in contrast to "independent providers" who work directly for elders or their families and are paid by the elders, their families, private insurance, or public benefits programs.

The term *predator* refers to people who actively seek out elders to exploit or assault. Financial predators range from petty con artists who take jobs at senior centers to gain access to potential victims, to highly sophisticated criminals. In the case of mass-marketing fraud, such as telemarketing fraud and identity theft, some perpetrators are believed to have ties to organized crime and terrorist groups (Binational Working Group on Cross-Border Mass-Marketing Fraud, 2003). Sexual predators include "gerophiles" or "gerontophiles," who have sexual inclinations toward the elderly (Kaul & Duffy, 1991; Ramsey-Klawsnik, 2004). Some seek employment at long-term care facilities or other "victim-rich" settings.

A cause for concern in recent years stems from the fact that sexual predators are also increasingly becoming nursing home residents (A Perfect Cause, 2005; Myers & Jacobo, 2005; U.S. Government Accountability Office, 2006). A survey by the Government Accountability Office (2006) found about 700 registered sex offenders living in long-term care facilities during 2005. Most identified sex offenders were male and under the age of sixty-five. About 3% of nursing homes housed at least one identified sex offender during 2005.

Other perpetrators of abuse in long-term care facilities include direct care workers and support staff, and temporary employees. Supervisors, management, or corporate entities may be responsible for abuse or neglect that results from inadequate staffing, supervision, or training (Morgan & Scott, 2003; Pillemer & Moore, 1989). Residents may also be abused by other residents, family members, and visitors. Perpetrators also include professionals and businesses. Professionals such as accountants, lawyers, and health care professionals are in particularly advantageous positions to gain access to elderly clients, and there are many bogus or unscrupulous businesses that target vulnerable elders.

Table 4.3 provides examples of perpetrators' characteristics that should be considered in developing service plans.

Perpetrator Characteristics that Affect Service Needs

Perpetrators' relationships to their victims are of particular importance in service planning because the relationship may determine whether reporting, criminal, and civil laws apply. For example, as described in Chapter 2, definitions of elder abuse used in reporting laws may only cover abuse that is committed by people who are in positions of trust or confidence with their victims such as family members, paid caregivers, family caregivers, friends, acquaintances, and professionals. Domestic violence laws typically offer protection to victims who are abused by spouses, intimate partners, estranged partners, and, in some jurisdictions, adult children or other family members. In addition, legal sanctions may be available when neglectful caregivers have a duty, by virtue of being a family member, to provide care.

Perpetrators' relationships to their victims also affect whether victims are willing to take steps to stop the abuse. When perpetrators are family members or friends, victims may refuse to take actions such as evicting

Table 4.3   Characteristics of Perpetrators

Perpetrators' Characteristics	Associated Risk Factors
Relationship to victims	• 90% of perpetrators are family members (National Center on Elder Abuse, 1998). • While household surveys show that spouses are most likely to abuse (Pillemer & Finkelhor, 1988; Podnieks, 1992), abuse by adult children is reported most often (National Center on Elder Abuse, 1998; Teaster, Dugar, Mendiondo, Abner, & Cecil, 2006). • 60% of APS-substantiated financial abuse cases are committed by adult children (National Center on Elder Abuse, 1998). • 42% of elder murders are committed by offspring, and 24% are by spouses (Dawson & Langan, 1994). • Perpetrators of homicide-suicide are typically male spouses or intimate partners (Cohen, 1998).
Mental health and behavioral problems	• Perpetrators are likely to have mental health, substance abuse, and behavioral problems (Anetzberger, 2005; Anetzberger, Korbin, & Austin, 1994; Greenberg et al., 1990; Lachs & Pillemer, 1995; Pillemer & Finkelhor, 1988; Wolf & Pillemer, 1989). • Abusers are likely to have histories of violence or antisocial behavior in other contexts outside the family (Lachs & Pillemer, 1995). • Abusive family caregivers are more likely than nonabusive ones to suffer from depression (Coyne, Reichman, & Berbig, 1993; Homer & Gilleard, 1990; Paveza et al., 1992). • Sexual assault by family members is often associated with mental health or substance abuse problems (Teaster & Roberto, 2004). • Employees in long-term care facilities who engage in physical and psychological abuse are likely to be experiencing "burnout," (progressive physical and emotional exhaustion resulting from prolonged involvement with people) (Hawes, 2003). • Perpetrators of homicide-suicide are likely to suffer from untreated and undetected psychiatric problems, especially depression (Cohen, 1998).
Dependency	• Adult children who abuse their elderly parents are likely to be unemployed, unmarried, and dependent on their victims emotionally, financially, and for housing (Anetzberger, 1987; Lachs and Pillemer, 1995; Pillemer & Finkelhor, 1988; Wolf, 1997).

Table 4.3 (*Continued*)

Perpetrators' Characteristics	Associated Risk Factors
Age	• Male abusers tend to be younger than their victims (National Center on Elder Abuse, 1998).
	• Abusive employees in long-term care facilities are younger than nonabusers and more likely to have negative attitudes about residents (Pillemer & Moore, 1990).
Gender	• Just over half (52.5%) of abusers are men for all forms of abuse.
	• Men are significantly more likely than women to commit certain types of abuse: abandonment (83%), physical abuse (63%), emotional abuse (60%), financial/material exploitation (59%) (National Center on Elder Abuse, 1998).
	• Nearly all perpetrators of suicide/homicides are men (Cohen, 2000).

them from their homes, severing contact, or taking punitive action out of guilt or loyalty. Elders who depend on their abusers for care or financial support may fear that reporting them will result in their becoming homeless or indigent. Some only agree to take action if their perpetrators receive needed help. This is particularly true when the abusers are troubled sons or daughters. As Dundorf and Brownell (1995) point out, "Practice experience and studies have demonstrated that victims often will not accept services for themselves if services are not also offered to their abusers." Successfully intervening in these cases may involve working with perpetrators as well as abusers or helping victims understand how counterproductive relationships can be.

The nature of the relationship between perpetrators and victims also determines what services and interventions are available and likely to be effective. For example, because of the highly charged nature of intimate relationships, interventions aimed at stopping domestic violence focus on protecting victims' safety (e.g., restraining orders, shelters, safety planning). In fact, many domestic violence advocates contend that interventions like mediation or couples counseling are inappropriate and dangerous in domestic violence because disparities in power between victims and abusers can lead to intimidation and/or further abuse.

In the case of abuse by caregivers, the nature of the caregiving relationship also dictates what can be done and what victims are willing to do. When paid caregivers who work for agencies commit abuse or neglect, they may be fired, disciplined, or provided with additional training or supervision. Elders who have hired caregivers independently can also fire workers, give them warnings, report them to the police if the abuse is criminal, or initiate lawsuits to recoup misappropriated assets.

Many victims, however, are unwilling to terminate their abusers' employment or report them to authorities. Some fear retaliation. And, owing to a critical shortage of caregivers, others fear that they will not be able to find replacements and will therefore have to make due without needed care or go into long-term care facilities. If a paid caregiver is a family member, the elder victim may not want to see the person lose his or her source of income. They may depend on the person for emotional support. Finally, caregivers may pressure or coerce victims into not reporting them or play upon their trust, sympathy, or loneliness.

Perpetrators' Reasons or Motives for Abusing

Many researchers have offered explanations for why abuse occurs. Although it is beyond the scope of this book to present or evaluate these explanations, a brief summary of commonly cited reasons or motives associated with abuse and neglect, and their implications for practice, is presented below.

- **Financial gain.** As more is learned about elder abuse, financial gain is increasingly being recognized as a primary motive not only for financial abuse, but for other forms of abuse as well, including neglect, intimidation, physical abuse, and homicide. For example, caregivers may deprive elders of needed care to make them more compliant or susceptible to undue influence, or they may attempt to hasten the elder's death if they stand to benefit. Similarly, physical abuse and psychological abuse may be motivated by financial gain.
- **Mental health problems.** Many perpetrators have mental illnesses, personality disorders, substance abuse problems, or dementias. Developmentally disabled adult children who have been cared for by their parents may be incapable of reciprocating when their parents need care (Anetzberger, 1987; Lachs & Pillemer, 1995; National Research Council, 2003).
- **Problems associated with caregiving.** Caregivers may abuse or neglect those they care for because they are under severe stress, exhausted, inexperienced, or reluctant to perform the caregiving role. They may lack skills, empathy, or understanding (Reis & Nahmiash, 1998). For example, they may think that an elder who is difficult to care for "is doing it on purpose." As described in Chapter 3, the emerging research on caregiving and elder abuse suggests the importance of such factors as disturbing behaviors by care receivers, the quality of "premorbid relationships" (prior

to the onset of disability), and mutual aggression as risk factors for caregiver abuse and neglect (Cooney & Mortimer, 1995).

- **Dependency.** Perpetrators are likely to be dependent on the people they abuse. In some cases, abuse results from attempts by relatives (especially adult offspring) to obtain resources from their victims, or there may be tensions because financially dependent sons or daughters are unwilling to leave and lose parental support. Adult children who abuse their elderly parents are likely to be unemployed, unmarried, and dependent on their victims (Lachs & Pillemer, 1995; Pillemer & Finkelhor, 1988; Wolf & Pillemer, 1989). The relationships between some perpetrators and victims have been described as a "mutual web of dependency," wherein victims depend on their abusers for care, and abusers depend on their victims for financial or emotional support and housing (Wolf & Pillemer, 1989).
- **Interpersonal dysfunction or unresolved conflict.** Abusers may abuse out of resentment, jealousy, or as retribution for actual or perceived wrongs committed against them by their victims or others.
- **Power and control.** The drive for power and control prompts some perpetrators, including perpetrators of domestic violence, to subjugate and subordinate their partners.

In assessing perpetrators' relationships with their victims and their reasons for abusing, workers need to consider the following:

- Does the nature of the relationship qualify victims for specialized services or protections (e.g., domestic violence services if the abuser is an intimate partner or family member)?
- Does the caregiver have a "duty" to provide care (e.g., are abusers paid to provide services or covered under laws requiring them to provide care or support)?
- What does the victim want with respect to the abuser? For example, does he or she want to sever all contact, see that the person gets help, etc?
- Is the victim dependent on the abuser for care, a place to live, and/ or emotional or financial support? Is the perpetrator dependent on the victim?
- Is the offender exercising power, control, or undue influence over the victim?

Abusers' Willingness and Ability to Change

The response of abusers regarding their willingness to change varies widely. Some abusers agree to stop abusing, assume responsibility for their actions, participate in treatment, or make amends out of remorse, shame, guilt, or because they have gained new insights or skills. Others respond to pressure or coercive techniques such as court-ordered counseling, mediation, restitution, or community service. Others deny responsibility for their actions or feel no remorse. They may not "buy into" society's code of conduct or deny what they did was wrong. Abusers who deny or minimize abuse are not likely to voluntarily stop the abuse or engage in therapeutic interventions. And finally, some abusers are unable to change their conduct as a result of mental illnesses, dementias, or developmental disabilities.

Abusers' willingness and ability to stop abusing or engage in treatment determines what interventions and services are available and appropriate for both abusers and victims. Abusers who are willing and able to change may be offered opportunities to make amends and/or engage in treatment in lieu of, or in addition to, punishment. Abusers' willingness and ability to stop abusing further determines whether their victims need ongoing protection, alternate caregivers or housing, and other services. In assessing perpetrators, workers should consider the following:

- What do victims want to see happen to their abusers?
- Are abusers willing and able to stop abuse, learn new skills, or participate in treatment?
- Does the offender admit to the wrongdoing and assume responsibility for it?
- Has the perpetrator paid back victims for property or assets?
- If offenders are being treated for mental illness, substance abuse, or other addictions (including gambling), can their progress and compliance be monitored?
- What protective, preventative, or support services do victims need to ensure their ongoing safety, security, and well-being in the event that perpetrators are unwilling or unable to stop abusing or break their promises to do so?

Abusers' Access and Level of Threat to Victims and Their Assets

In developing service plans, workers and victims need to take into account the immediacy of the threat that perpetrators pose. When abusers have continued access to elders and their belongings, interventions must focus on victims' safety and security. Services that may be needed include shelter, safety plans, and restraining orders. When perpetrators have access to elders' bank accounts or other financial documents, or have assumed elders' identities, immediate action may be needed to preserve and recover assets and stop further harm.

Even when abusers do not pose an immediate threat (e.g., they have vacated victims' homes, moved away, or been incarcerated), future risk should be anticipated. For example, victims can ask to be notified of incarcerated abusers' release dates. APS and other aging service providers are increasingly working with corrections, probation, and parole personnel to monitor abusers and ensure victim safety and security. Even when perpetrators have willingly agreed to or have been court-ordered into treatment programs, they may still pose a threat. Therefore, those working with victims need to be attentive to potential danger. Family members, friends, service providers, and others may be enlisted to help monitor situations with clients' consent. And finally, it must be noted that victims may be willing to accept the risk of ongoing contact.

The danger that perpetrators pose to their victims and potential victims also dictates the extent to which they are allowed to maintain contact, continue providing help, be given second chances, and participate in treatment.

Specific questions to consider include the following:

- Does the offender pose a threat to the victim's safety?
- Does he or she have access to the victim or his or her property?
- Will the offender have access to the victim in the future?
- Does the offender have access to other vulnerable elders?
- Are there factors that mitigate the dangerousness or risk of future abuse? For example, are others present in victims' homes who can monitor situations or have victims' assets been secured?

URGENCY OF THE SITUATION

A critical consideration in determining what services and interventions are needed is whether abusers pose an immediate or imminent risk to victims' safety, health, or property. In urgent or emergency situations, aggressive measures may be available that are not available under other circumstances. For example, protective custody and mental health hospitalizations may be warranted when victims or others are in imminent danger. Similarly, interventions to seize and freeze assets may only be available when there is an imminent threat of loss (see Chapter 5). Special emergency measures may also be needed to ensure that perpetrators are caught, do not harm others, or destroy property or evidence. Because these emergency measures may significantly restrict clients' or perpetrators' autonomy, they should be used judiciously.

Examples of emergencies and urgent situations include the following:

- When elders who require supervision are left alone. They may, for example, have suffered accidents, injuries, or decline that renders them unable to meet their own needs. Or their caregivers may have abandoned them, been fired or arrested, died, or become incapable of providing adequate care.
- When elders are in imminent danger of violence or physical injury. For example, they have been threatened.
- When violent offenders have access to potential new victims.
- When elders are about to be evicted for nonpayment of rent, noncompliance with the terms of their tenancy, and so on.
- When elder's homes, residences, or physical environment are unsafe.
- When elders are at imminent risk of serious financial losses. For example, a victim with diminished capacity has signed a bank power of attorney naming an abuser as attorney in fact and there is money in the account.

In assessing the need for emergency responses, workers need to consider the following:

- What is at risk?
- How great is the risk?
- What emergency interventions are available?

ETHICAL CONSIDERATIONS

In deciding how to intervene in abuse cases, service providers are also guided by their professional orientation and values. Although there are no universally accepted ethical principles for practice in the field of elder abuse prevention, many APS workers subscribe to those developed by the National Adult Protective Services Association. The National Association of Social Workers, the American Medical Association, and other professional organizations have also developed codes of ethics for their members. There is, however, general agreement that autonomy, self-determination, and least restrictive alternatives are among the principles that form the basic ethical framework for practice in the field.

Autonomy and Self-Determination

Autonomy refers to people's right to make decisions for themselves that are voluntary and free from interference by others. The closely related concept of self-determination refers to people's ability to manage their own affairs, make their own judgments, and provide for themselves. Applying these principles to elder abuse prevention requires workers to abide by clients' wishes with respect to intervening or not intervening, and their choices with respect to services. Workers can help enhance their clients' autonomy by providing them with tools, information, and assistance and by removing threats to autonomy and self-determination such as coercion, duress, and undue influence.

Even when elders lack the capacity needed to make decisions, those advocating for them or making decisions on their behalf should still respect the elders' autonomy to the greatest extent possible. The following hierarchy of approaches is generally accepted:

- Honor preferences that the person has expressed in the past before the onset of incapacity. These can be determined by consulting clients' records and people who know them.
- If preferences are not known, surrogates use "substituted judgment." This means that decisions are based on what the person would have wanted or preferred. This approach requires substantial information about clients' views and wishes.
- When there is insufficient information on which to base substituted judgment, surrogates must decide based on their judgment about what would be in the "best interest" of the client. Judgments should be based on what a rational, normal person would prefer, not just on what the surrogate prefers.
- In cases in which physicians, surrogates, other family members, service providers, or other legitimately involved persons disagree about what is in the person's best interest, parties should be encouraged and provided with opportunities to meet and exchange information and views.
- In cases where agreement cannot be reached, interested parties should consult ethics committees if available. Other options include consulting with multidisciplinary elder abuse teams or other problem-solving groups. When surrogates or physicians are acting against the expressed preferences or best interests of patients, courts may need to be consulted.

Least Restrictive Alternatives

APS workers and others also operate on the principle that priority should be given to interventions that least restrict clients' autonomy, independence, and freedom of choice.

The concept of least restrictive alternatives emerged from the field of mental health during the 1970s when advocates sought less restrictive alternatives to institutionalizing people with mental illnesses. It has been widely applied and adapted by other disciplines in other settings. For example, long-term care options fall along a continuum with home-based services being on the least restrictive end and skilled nursing homes on the most restrictive. Similarly, there is a continuum of options available for people who are having difficulty managing their finances, which range from informal money management to guardianship of estate. The "least restrictive" principle has also been applied to specific interventions. For example, judges are encouraged to craft "limited guardianships" whenever possible, permitting wards to retain as much choice and autonomy as possible (ABA, APA, & National College of Probate Judges, 2006).

Other Ethical Principles

Other ethical principles that may apply in elder abuse cases include the following:

- Beneficence: The obligation to do good and assist others further their interests
- Justice: The fair and equitable distribution of benefits and burdens. For protective and social service workers, this includes ensuring that their clients have equitable access to service resources
- Nonmaleficence: It is morally wrong to harm others. Because helping others often requires the infliction of a lesser harm in order to avoid a major imminent harm, nonmaleficence is generally taken to mean "Do not cause other persons to die, suffer pain or disability, or deprive them of their most important interests, unless you have a good reason."
- Privacy: The right of individuals to keep their lives and personal affairs out of public view, or to control information about themselves.
- The benefits over burden standard. This standard is often applied when questions arise about whether or not treatment is indicated. It presumes that the benefits of treatment to peoples' quality of life should outweigh the burdens they impose.

Competing and Conflicting Principles

Elder abuse cases often raise troubling ethical issues. For instance, ethical principles may conflict with legal mandates, as is the case when workers are required to report abuse to authorities against their clients' wishes. Adhering to certain ethical principles may arouse controversy or criticism from third parties, as is often the case when workers defend their clients' autonomy by honoring their wishes to remain in unsafe situations. Ethical principles may also be in conflict with cultural values. For example, some cultures place greater value on group well-being than the well-being of individuals (see the following section for more about this). In fact, some have gone so far as to suggest that self-determination is a white, middle-class value, which does not serve the best interests of cultural groups that value group well-being above individual desires or self-gain (Bergeron, 1999). Even attitudes about privacy are culturally determined; the common practice of interviewing clients privately may be viewed with suspicion within some cultural communities.

When workers are faced with ethical dilemmas or conflicts, they can benefit from soliciting input from supervisors and peers. Some communities also have ethics committees, although most ethics committees are convened by hospitals and nursing homes and focus on medical decisions. However, there appears to be growing interest in developing ethics committees that address ethical issues that arise in the community. Multidisciplinary teams can also provide a forum for discussing ethical issues. Discussing cases with others also provides workers with an opportunity to ensure that they are acting in accordance with the accepted values of their communities and professions. This may be important to demonstrate if their actions are ever questioned.

Ethical considerations that should be taken into account in working with elder abuse clients include the following:

- To what extent are clients able to exercise autonomy and self-determination? How can their ability to do so be maximized?
- Have elders with diminished capacity expressed their preferences in the past? Are their wishes known?
- Are there less restrictive alternatives to those being considered? What are the benefits and risks of each?
- Are there conflicts with respect to ethical issues?

CULTURAL FACTORS AFFECTING SERVICE NEEDS

The cultural context in which abuse occurs also dictates service needs. Cultural factors affect what conduct is seen as abusive within various communities, attitudes about what should be done about it, what services are acceptable, and obstacles to accessing services. Cultural factors further influence attitudes about the social service and legal systems. Cultural bonds and institutions can also be a valuable resource, supplementing and enhancing formal services by providing social, emotional, and spiritual support.

Culture refers to the experiences, values, language, and customs shared by people of the same ethnicity, race, or background. Shared experiences may also include immigration, racism, the pressures of acculturation, economic hurdles, and history. These factors have a significant impact on family life, including members' relationships, expectations, and conduct toward each other. Although every cultural community is unique, and it is well beyond the scope of this chapter to summarize the emergent literature on abuse and neglect in diverse communities, this section introduces some of the cultural factors that have been explored as they relate to service needs. Hopefully, it can serve as a template to help service providers explore the specific attributes and needs of those they serve. For those who want to learn more, there are several excellent resources that can serve as starting points, including Toshio Tatara's *Understanding Elder Abuse in Minority Populations,* and the Clearinghouse on Abuse and Neglect of the Elderly's (CANE) *Annotated Bibliography on Cultural Issues in Elder Abuse.*[2]

Cultural Factors Affecting Risk

Although the literature on cultural variations in elder abuse has proceeded slowly, patterns are apparent with respect to the frequency and severity of various forms of abuse within specific communities. For example, a 2003 study by the Federal Trade Commission revealed that certain racial and ethnic minorities were much more likely to be victims of fraud, including telemarketing scams, then whites. Nearly 34% of American Indians and Alaska Natives, 17% of African Americans, and over 14% of Hispanics had experienced one or more frauds in the preceding year compared to just over 6% for whites (Federal Trade Commission, 2004).

Cultural factors also affect risk. As noted earlier, living together is among the most significant risk factors for elder abuse (Pillemer & Finkelhor, 1988). Black, Hispanic, and Asian and Pacific Islander elders are much more likely than whites to live with family members other than spouses (Administration on Aging, 2004), potentially raising their risk. In addition, adult children, grandchildren, and other family members may move into elders' home due to stressful life events such as divorce or unemployment, further contributing to risk (Benton, 1998). The risk may, however, be mitigated by the support and security that multigenerational families can offer.

Caregivers also have more demands placed upon them within some communities of color. The adult children of African American and Native American seniors, for example, provide significantly more hours of care and higher-intensity care than whites, and are likely to provide care to multiple members, including minor grandchildren and extended family members (Baldridge & Benson, 2005; Figueroa, 2003; Griffin & Williams, 1992; Hargrave, 2006; Nerenberg & Njeri, 1993). Elders within these communities are generally in poorer health than whites and are likely to have illnesses and disabling conditions like diabetes that create particularly heavy demands on caregivers (National Institute on Aging, 2006). Furthermore, the lack of culturally appropriate nursing homes, or nursing homes in general for these communities, may lead families to provide care beyond the point that it is reasonable to do so.

Many of the factors that have been suggested as contributing to the risk of abuse are associated with poverty, which disproportionately affects minorities, and, to an even greater extent, women (Hounsell & Riojas, 2006). Poverty-related factors that have been suggested as contributing to risk include health status (described above), poor nutritional status, substandard housing, isolation, lack of access to services and care, and higher rates of mental health problems, including depression, substance abuse, low self-esteem, and a sense of powerlessness and hopelessness about the future (Simpson, 2005; Tatara, 1999). However, there has been little research on the direct relationship between poverty and elder abuse, with one notable exception being a study that compared an impoverished Plains Indian reservation with a wealthier one. The study found significantly less abuse on the wealthier reservation (Maxwell & Maxwell, 1992).

Changing values within cultural communities can also lead to strife and the loss of cultural cohesion (Baldridge, 2002; Stanford, 1998; Torres-Gil, 1998). Within immigrant and marginalized communities, there is often intense pressure to "acculturate" to mainstream culture. According to Fernando Torres-Gil, Ph.D., dean of academic affairs at the School of Public Policy and Social Work at the University of California, Los Angeles, "Elder abuse is a manifestation of the pressures falling on Hispanic families today. Traditionally, Hispanics have venerated their elders. But this is changing . . . We're starting to see ageism and individualism corrupt our community" (Torres-Gil, 1998).

Other experts have pointed out that cultural forces can also mitigate the risk of elder abuse and neglect. These include cultural traditions that hold elders in high esteem and "filial piety" or "filial responsibility," which refer to adult children's obligation toward their aging parents, which includes providing financial and emotional support, and housing (Pinquart & Sörensen, 2005; Tatara, 1999; Tomita, 1994). The specific roles and obligations of adult children toward their parents vary by culture, and even within cultural groups. For example, children's responsibilities toward parents may be determined by gender and birth order (Montgomery & Kosloski, 2000).

Interdependency, which is also highly valued within many cultural communities, can contribute to elderly members' well-being and security

(Montoya, 1997; Rittman, Kuzmeskus, & Flum, 1999). Speaking about African American families, Donna Benton (1998) points out, "Multigenerational family units provide support and stability to members, and the sharing of family homes and resources has allowed families to subsist on minimal incomes." In describing elderly Navajos' attitudes about elder abuse, Arnold Brown observed that "At the heart of their traditional culture was that family members had the obligation to relate to each other in interdependency and mutually share what they had, with no thought given to the idea that they had any rights as individuals." This extended to the common practice of sharing their SSI or Social Security checks out of a sense of duty to their families (Brown, 1998).

Attitudes about Abuse

Just as cultural factors influence risk, cultural values and expectations affect how members perceive abuse and neglect (Brown, 1999; Moon & Williams, 1993; Simpson, 2005). For example, as described earlier, within some Native American families, using an elder's public benefits or pension for the benefit of other family members is viewed as the appropriate sharing of resources, whereas outsiders may see it as exploitation (Brown, 1999; Hudson & Carlson, 1999). Similarly, many elderly Koreans believe that it is acceptable for husbands to restrict wives' access to their families' financial resources (Moon & Williams, 1993). And, within the African American community, placing elders in nursing homes is often perceived as an act of abuse (Patterson & Malley-Morrison, 2006).

Culture further dictates what types of abuse are seen as most serious. For example, Caucasian elders are more tolerant of verbal abuse than Korean Americans, whereas Korean Americans are more tolerant of financial exploitation (Moon & Williams, 1993).

Obstacles to Accessing Services

Culture variations also exist among groups with respect to the likelihood that members will seek out and accept help, what types of help are acceptable, and service needs. For example, some studies indicate that older adults of Asian or Hispanic descent prefer turning to family or friends for assistance, whereas African Americans are more likely to turn to formal service providers or the police (Anetzberger, 1998; Anetzberger, Korbin, & Tomita, 1996; Moon & Williams, 1993). The reasons for these decisions may vary. Members of marginalized groups may not want to reveal conduct that exposes their communities to scrutiny or reflects poorly on them, or it may be considered disloyal to reveal problems to outsiders.

Cultural factors further influence what services are viewed as acceptable. Certain forms of medical care and social services are viewed as abusive by members of some cultural groups (Lachs & Pillemer, 2004), and members of marginalized communities are particularly likely to have negative attitudes about the criminal justice system (Shipler, Anand, & Hadi, 1998). Immigrant victims may not be willing to report if they come from countries where police brutality or corruption is common, and undocumented victims may not contact police or social service agencies for fear of being deported or seeing their abusers deported.

And finally, "mainstream" services may not meet the needs of members of cultural communities. For example, nearly three-fourths of African-American and Hispanic caregivers are adult children, whereas the majority of white caregivers are spouses (Montgomery & Kosloski, 2000). The needs of caregiving children tend to differ from those of spousal caregivers, for whom most caregiving services are geared. For example, caregiving daughters who work are more likely to need programs like adult day care centers that operate during working hours, whereas spouses typically prefer in-home services that allow them short breaks to get out (Hargrave, 2006; Pinquart & Sörensen, 2005). Other obstacles that members of cultural communities face in accessing abuse prevention services include the lack of culturally appropriate and language-appropriate services. Service providers' attitudes about clients whose cultural backgrounds are different from their own may also create barriers. For example, commonly held beliefs that certain groups "take care of their own" may lead service providers to the mistaken conclusion that elders do not need formal supports.

Cultural Considerations Affecting Practice

In working with clients from diverse communities, workers are encouraged to learn as much as possible about those they serve. Asking clients, family members, or colleagues questions in a respectful way is generally acceptable and appreciated.

Questions to consider include the following:

- How are elders and aging viewed?
- How is abuse viewed within the community (what types of conduct are seen as abusive, what are the causes, how serious is it, and what should be done about it?)
- What cultural factors contribute to or mitigate risk?
- Are there economic, social, or historical factors that prevent seniors from accessing "mainstream" services?
- What formal and informal supports exist within the community?

CONCLUSION

No two cases of abuse or neglect are quite alike. Cases, therefore, need to be looked at individually to determine clients' needs using the criteria described in this chapter and others.

A variety of assessment tools exist that can provide additional guidance, which are described in Chapter 5. Although these tools provide a good starting point, professionals are essentially on their own when it comes to matching clients to promising interventions. Because few services and interventions have been evaluated, little is known about their effectiveness, and even less is known about the value of various services for specific client groups. For example, little is known about the effectiveness of services for elders with mild or moderate cognitive impairments and elders from diverse cultural communities. In addition, when resources are inadequate, which is often the case, workers have to use whatever is available.

These obstacles may well explain the popularity of multidisciplinary case review teams, which provide a dynamic process and forum for professionals from diverse disciplines to explore potential interventions on a case-by-case basis and customize service plans to meet clients' specific needs. Multidisciplinary teams and how they work are explained in Chapter 6.

NOTES

1. The National Research Council's 2003 publication *Elder Mistreatment: Abuse, Neglect, and Exploitation in an Aging America* provides an analysis of elder abuse risk factors.
2. Available at Available at http://www.ncea.aoa.gov/NCEAroot/Main_Site/Library/CANE/CANE_Series/CANE_cultural.aspx.

CHAPTER FIVE

Preventing and Treating Elder Abuse

INTRODUCTION

Choosing a format for this chapter, which describes elder abuse prevention services and interventions, was challenging. Other books and articles have been organized in a variety of ways—from the sequencing of interventions, to listing interventions in relation to specific forms of abuse, to describing methods used by various disciplines.

But elder abuse and its treatment defy simple schemas. The focal point of interventions may shift between victims and abusers, multiple forms of abuse often occur simultaneously, and there is no single point of entry into the service system. In other words, cases do not conform to uniform patterns, and layers of complexity continually unfold.

I have, therefore, compromised with an approach that borrows from many of my predecessors. I have begun with a description of assessment because it is often the first step in intervening; however, assessment is an ongoing process, and workers continually assess clients' needs and revise care plans accordingly throughout the intervention process. Services for victims come next and are organized by the goals they attempt to achieve, which include (1) maximizing independence; (2) resolving crises and emergencies; (3) ensuring victim safety; (4) healing, empowering, and supporting victims; (5) preserving, protecting, and recovering assets; and (6) ensuring justice. The remaining sections focus on interventions with perpetrators and those at risk for abusing.

This chapter is not a step-by-step guide or protocol. Rather, it simply describes interventions and services used in the field. In some cases, I have sought the help of colleagues to provide a clearer view of the what, when, how, and whys of what they do. And, where available, I have provided information about the effectiveness of services and interventions.

The services and interventions described here may be provided by APS; other public agencies; private, nonprofit agencies; and for-profit agencies and organizations. Some are offered by church groups or advocacy organizations. Unfortunately, many are not yet available in all or even most communities. I encourage readers to stay apprised of local resources by participating in elder abuse prevention coalitions or multidisciplinary teams. The National Center on Elder Abuse's Web site also describes promising practices in the field.[1]

ASSESSING VICTIMS' SERVICE NEEDS

From the moment that professionals suspect or are informed of abuse, they start making judgments. The trigger may be a telltale indicator they observe themselves, or calls from concerned neighbors, family members, colleagues, or, occasionally, victims. Although APS workers, law enforcement, and LTC Ombudsmen are the most likely "first responders"; others, including case managers, medical personnel, employees of senior centers, health care facilities, or even banks, may be the first to discover or suspect abuse and neglect.

Among the initial judgments that professionals make is whether or not to drop what they are doing to make immediate home visits or gather additional information. They must determine if the elder is in immediate danger or why someone has chosen now to call. In other words, they triage cases. As workers gather information, they continue to make judgments, assessing whether elders are able to manage on their own, for how long, if they are capable of making decisions for themselves, and whether they are being coerced or unduly influenced by others.

Seasoned workers become highly skilled at making these judgments. Some seem to know immediately and instinctively if abuse occurred or is likely to and how serious it is. Using the lens of experience, they evaluate what they are seeing or being told, weigh it against what they have learned from past experience and clients, and use the information to decide what course of action to take.

But for most workers, elder abuse cases are daunting. Situations aren't always what they appear to be at first blush, and many victims deny that they have been abused or are at risk. Some downplay what has happened, whereas others overstate it. It is not surprising that APS workers and others have identified assessment as one of the most difficult aspects of their work.

Assessment is the formal process for evaluating clients' situations, conditions, and service needs. Assessments are typically carried out during the early stages of case planning and repeated at intervals to identify changes and new needs. In elder abuse cases, the process of assessment involves evaluating clients' overall well-being, health status, ability to manage independently, and decision-making capacity as well as their level of risk, the type of abuse they are at risk for, its seriousness, and the potential consequences. All of these factors dictate the client's needs.

Formal assessment can accomplish other important objectives as well. Assessment tools provide a mechanism for monitoring changes over time, alert workers to impending or early stage problems, and suggest whether interventions are effective. Assessment tools also provide objective measures so clients can be compared and prioritized.

In addition, aggregate information drawn from assessments is valuable to researchers and practitioners in helping them understand risk factors, patterns, trends, and clients themselves. It also provides program managers and supervisors information on which to base management decisions with respect to allocating resources, determining caseload size, and determining workers' effectiveness.

Specifically, assessment can accomplish the following:

- Determine whether elders are able to manage on their own
- Determine what services are needed
- Identify, evaluate, and document risk factors and indicators that suggest that abuse has occurred or is likely to
- Alert workers to crises
- Prioritize cases
- Help managers to evaluate workers' performance, assign cases equitably, and allocate resources
- Develop a baseline of information that can be compared over time
- Determine whether interventions and services have been successful by indicating changes in the severity or duration of symptoms or risk factors over time
- Increase knowledge about abuse

A wide variety of assessment tools are currently in use. Among the most popular "functional assessment tools," which measure people's ability to meet their own needs, are the Activities of Daily Living (ADL) and Instrumental Activities of Daily Living (IADL) scales (Gallo, 2006). The ADL scale measures people's ability to perform a variety of personal care tasks such as bathing, eating, dressing, getting in and out of bed and chairs, using the toilet, and walking. The IADL scale measures more complicated tasks like the ability to balance checkbooks, perform housework, go grocery shopping, prepare meals, arrange for outside services, drive or take public transportation, manage finances, and take medications.

Cognitive assessment tools measure the mental skills people use to perform mental tasks. They range from simple screening tools that suggest problems and the need for more detailed analyses, to comprehensive batteries of tests that must be administered by highly trained professionals. Perhaps the most commonly used screening tool is the Mini-Mental State Examination (Folstein, Folstein, & McHugh, 1975), which covers memory, language, spatial ability, and set-shifting. It is relatively easy to administer and is commonly used by APS workers, case managers, and physicians. The results, however, are imperfect and should only be used as a rough indicator to determine if and when more thorough assessment is needed. The Repeatable Battery for the Assessment of Neuropsychological Status is another screening tool that is used to detect and characterize dementia in the elderly. It measures attention, language, visuospatial/constructional abilities, and immediate and delayed memory (Randolph, 1998). The Executive Interview (EXIT 25) identifies signs of impaired executive control functioning that are believed by some to be a risk factor for financial abuse (Royall, Mahurin, & Gray, 1992). Another commonly used and simple to administer tool to screen for impaired executive function, language and verbal fluency, and early Alzheimer's disease is the "Animal Naming Test" in which patients are asked to name as many animals as they can in one minute.

More comprehensive cognitive testing is advised when the outcome of the testing has serious implications (e.g., guardianship is being considered). "Dementia workups," which are usually performed by physicians, help determine the cause of dementia-like symptoms and identify "pseudo dementias" that may be treatable or reversible (e.g., delirium, depression, substance abuse, malnutrition, metabolic disorders, urinary tract infections, and neurological diseases) (Kane, Ouslander, & Abrass, 1994). Neuropsychological testing, which is typically conducted by clinical psychologists, may be needed when clients have capabilities in some areas but not others and there is no clear explanation for the differences (Quinn & Tomita, 1997).

Risk assessment tools help determine if abuse or neglect have occurred or if elders are at risk (Johnson, 1991). Many tools have been created, and determining which ones are appropriate for specific clients or situations depends on a variety of factors including the setting, whether abuse is known to have occurred (or is only suspected), and its seriousness. For example, the American Medical Association recommends that doctors routinely ask all their elderly patients a few simple screening questions even if there are no signs or symptoms (American Medical Association, 1992). Other, more detailed assessments are needed when allegations have been made.

Risk assessment tools may be administered at various times during the investigation and care planning process (e.g., during the initial assessment, periodically while cases are open, and at case closure). Commonly used tools include the Elder Abuse and Neglect Assessment (Fulmer, 2003), the Hwalek & Sengstock Elder Abuse Screening Test (Neale, Hwalek, Scott, Sengstock, & Stahl, 1991), and the Indicators of Abuse Screen (Reis & Nahmiash, 1998).

Assessment tools generally contain lists of indicators or conditions that may be rated by severity, including the following (Wolf, 2000):

- Client factors such as age, gender, health, and confusion
- Environmental risk factors such as the condition of elders' homes and the absence of utilities
- Support services including the availability and adequacy of formal and informal support systems
- Current and historical abuse factors such as previous histories of abuse
- Abuser factors such as caregivers' mental health problems and caregiving skills

Risk assessment tools are highly controversial, and experts disagree about their effectiveness (Fulmer, Guadagno, Dyer, & Connolly, 2004; Wolf, 2000). Many workers find them cumbersome, and some fear that they may even have negative consequences such as exposing individuals or agencies to liability if they document risks and fail to effectively stop the problem.

Wolf (2000) notes that little progress has been made in quantifying or standardizing the process of risk assessment and that it is still basically a qualitative process that reflects clinical judgments as opposed to objective measures. In fact, few tools have been tested clinically to determine how accurate they are in either finding cases or predicting outcomes.

After comparing three common tools, Meeks-Sjostrom (2004) concluded that all have limitations and a new one should be developed. A governmental task force pointed out that the risks and benefits of assessment tools are impossible to determine when there are no studies that examine the effectiveness of interventions with victims (Nelson, Nygren, McInerney, & Klein, 2004; U.S. Preventive Task Force, 2004). And finally, Fulmer et al. (2003) emphasize the importance of "context" when assessing risk. When assessing neglect, for example, workers need to consider patients' and caregivers' health status, their socioeconomic and life circumstances, the credibility of the data collected by others, and the consequences of the assessment outcome (Fulmer et al., 2003).

Several specialized risk assessment tools have been developed to assess various types or aspects of elder abuse. These include the Risk of Elder Abuse in the Home (REAH) and the IDEAL protocol. The REAH scale alerts users to family strain and changes within family systems that heighten risk (Allison, Ellis, & Wilson, 1998; Hamilton, 1989). The IDEAL protocol, developed by forensic and geriatric psychiatrist Bennett Blum, describes psychological and social factors that commonly coexist in undue influence situations.[2] A "Self-neglect Severity Scale" is currently being developed by the Consortium for Research in Elder Self-neglect of Texas.[3]

Tools that are commonly used in other fields to assess the extent and consequences of violence are also increasingly being applied to elder abuse. These include "lethality assessment tools," which are primarily used in the field of domestic violence to predict future dangerousness (Websdale, 2000), and trauma assessments, which help to gauge victims' response to trauma. An example of a trauma assessment tool is the SPAN scale, which has been used to assess and document the impact of sexual assault on older women (Burgess & Clements, 2006).

Many agencies and states have drawn from standardized tools to design their own tools that combine functional and risk assessment measures. Some have developed highly specialized tools for specific purposes. For example, California's Forensic Medical Report: Elder and Dependent Adult Abuse and Neglect Examination form was designed to improve elder abuse documentation for legal purposes (Koin, 2003).

SERVICES AND INTERVENTIONS FOR VICTIMS

The services and interventions used with victims of elder abuse and neglect are designed to achieve many very specific objectives. To help make sense of these myriad objectives, I have divided them into the following overarching goals:

- Maximizing independence
- Resolving crises and emergencies
- Ensuring victim safety
- Healing, empowering, and supporting victims
- Preserving, protecting, and recovering assets
- Ensuring justice

Maximizing Independence

Experts acknowledge that the risk of elder abuse, neglect, self-neglect, and undue influence is heightened when elders are isolated, in poor health, and dependent on others for care. Conversely, risk can potentially be reduced by reducing isolation, improving overall physical and mental health and well-being, and promoting independence. These are the goals of support services and case management.

Support Services

Support services enable elders with disabilities to live independently in the community. These services include home delivered meals, attendant care, day programs, friendly visitors, transportation, telephone reassurance, home modification, and many others. In addition to promoting independence, these services can provide a "lifeline" to those who can be called upon for help. Service providers have also noted that offering support services is a good way to establish credibility and gain the trust and confidence of clients who are unwilling or reluctant to accept protective services or to take action against abusers.

Case Management

Case management is an approach to "brokering" or coordinating services for individuals who have multiple and changing care needs. Case managers conduct comprehensive assessments of clients' general health, mental capacity, and ability to manage in their homes and communities using functional and cognitive assessment tools like those described earlier. They then work with clients to develop "care plans," often in consultation with professionals from several disciplines, and arrange for services, respond to problems or emergencies, and conduct routine reassessments to detect changes.

Specialized case management has been designed to accommodate special needs. For example, mental health case management is for people with mental health problems, public health case management is for people who require monitoring for medical or health problems, and financial case managers have expertise in financial matters. Case managers are increasingly gaining expertise in working with abuse victims, who often require services that fall outside the scope of the traditional long-term care network. In fact, some professionals have called for the expanded use of case management in adult protective services (Cambridge & Parkes, 2004). Chapter 10 also argues for a more prominent role for case management in the field of elder abuse prevention.

Resolving Crises and Emergencies

Crises and emergencies are sudden changes, turning points, or unstable conditions that can be stressful or traumatic. Crises may be precipitated by physical or cognitive decline, financial losses, the death of loved ones or caregivers, or other traumatic events. Crises in the lives of elders may also be triggered by changes in the lives of their caregivers or family members, such as illnesses or financial setbacks that reduce the caregivers' ability to help. Crises may heighten elders' vulnerability to abuse or even trigger it.

Crises and emergencies pose special challenges. Even simple entry into an elder's residence during emergencies can be a problem when elders are alone and unable or unwilling to answer the door. Workers are likely to find clients in deteriorated states, injured, or traumatized. They must often intervene with very little background information on their clients. In addition, sometimes clients who are experiencing crises are unable or unwilling to accept help, participate in planning for their own care or safety, or even follow simple steps or directions. However, the consequences of not intervening may be great, and failure to intervene quickly may result in irreparable harm or loss. The goal in working with vulnerable and abused elders during crises and emergencies is to ensure their safety, reduce trauma, and secure assets.

Assessing Crises and Emergencies

Home visits are recommended in most crises and emergencies, and should be made as soon as possible (Quinn & Tomita, 1997). The most appropriate agency/individual to conduct home visits is determined by the community's protocols or guidelines for handling abuse referrals. In most communities, the agency charged with responding is APS.

When workers are unable to gain entrée in crises, they may need to get help from apartment managers, landlords, neighbors, family members, or the police (in many communities, police are authorized to conduct "well-being" or "welfare" checks on elders whose welfare is in question). Once inside the home, workers should assess whether elders are (1) responsive; (2) oriented to time, place, and person; (3) able to meet their own basic needs; and (4) able to obtain needed help.

Workers should also assess the nature and extent of the risk and whether immediate action is needed to prevent irreparable harm or loss. Questions to consider include the following:

- Does the elder need immediate medical attention or mental health care?

- Does the elder need to be removed from the home because it is unsafe to remain there (e.g., the home is extremely deteriorated or a violent offender is likely to return)?
- Do assets need to be secured?
- Are others at risk?
- Are formal or informal supports, such as family members, friends, attendants, or others available to provide assistance, support, or monitoring?

Crisis Counseling

Crisis counseling allows victims to express their reactions and reduces their emotional distress. Some studies show that giving people an opportunity to talk about their experiences very soon after a catastrophic event may reduce some of the symptoms of post-traumatic stress disorder (PTSD, National Institute of Mental Health, 2001). Descriptions of crisis counseling commonly describe the following techniques:

- Drawing from coping skills used in the past to respond to new challenges.
- Challenging irrational beliefs and unrealistic expectations.
- Creating temporary dependencies. During crises, even extremely capable people can become immobilized. Although the role of workers under ordinary circumstances is to foster independence, it may be appropriate to provide "hands on" help to clients (e.g., making calls for them) as long as the dependency is temporary.
- Helping people face fear, emotional pain, and sadness.
- Breaking "vicious cycles" and addictive behavior. Crises may trigger unhealthy escape through medications, drugs, and alcohol. These escape mechanisms need to be addressed.
- Helping victims understand their own behavior and that of others. Crisis intervention allows people to explore how they have contributed to crises and find alternatives.

Little is known about the special needs of elderly victims in crisis or the impact of crisis counseling. Among the few available studies is one that explored the use of crisis intervention with elderly victims of sexual assault (Tyra, 1996). Tyra observes that the focus of crisis intervention in sexual assault cases is to increase adaptive coping skills, regain equilibrium, and transition from being a "victim" to being a "survivor." Differences between elderly victims in crisis and their younger counterparts include the fact that elderly victims are more likely to have concerns about losing their independence and autonomy. Tyra emphasizes that helping elderly women in crisis make decisions and take action to resolve crises and improve the quality of their lives requires adequate time, empathic listening, the development of trust, and ongoing support.

Emergency Services

As described in Chapter 4, emergencies in elder abuse cases include situations in which elders who require supervision are left alone, when they are in imminent danger of violence or physical injury, when violent offenders have access to potential new victims, when elders' homes are in jeopardy or are unsafe, and when elders are at imminent risk of serious financial losses. Services that may be needed include emergency funds, emergency attendant care, shelter, psychiatric hospitalization or protective custody, emergency orders of protection, and emergency decision makers (including emergency guardians).

Emergency funds may be needed to pay for "basics" like food, utilities, transportation, or new locks to secure homes. Elders who are in danger of losing their homes as a result of eviction or foreclosure may need funds for rent or mortgage payments. Those living in unsafe homes may need to make repairs or modifications, or hire cleaning services. And those elders who need to move may need funds to cover relocation costs or security deposits. And finally, when cases are referred to courts, victims may need funds to cover attorneys' fees or court filing fees. Typically, emergency funds are maintained by APS programs or other health and human service providers (Nerenberg, 2000b).

Emergency in-home attendant care may be needed by elders who are unable to manage on their own if their caregivers abandon them, become incapacitated, or are terminated or arrested. Emergency attendants may serve as an alternative to shelter. To facilitate referrals, some APS programs have developed special contracts or memoranda of understanding with providers of attendant care, which describe how emergency referrals will be handled and paid for. Emergency attendants can also benefit from special training in abuse-related issues such as working with victims in crisis and the enforcement of orders of protection.

Psychiatric hospitalization may be needed by elderly victims who are gravely disabled or dangerous to themselves or others. Under state laws, certain professionals, including mental health workers, crisis teams, or police, are authorized to remove these individuals from their homes and admit them to psychiatric facilities for time-limited, involuntary treatment and evaluation. Typically, states' statutes only pertain to people who need to be hospitalized as a result of mental illnesses, although some states have extended coverage to people with dementias, nutritional deficiencies, and trauma who meet the other criteria.

A few states have created special provisions for "protective custody" for adults and elders who are incapacitated or gravely disabled for other reasons besides mental illness and/or who are at risk for abuse, neglect, or exploitation. Under these statutes, designated individuals may remove adults from their homes and place them in protective settings for short periods to assess their protective service needs. The goal is to remove the immediate risk, stabilize the situation, and determine whether the impairment is permanent or temporary. These statutes vary widely with respect to who can initiate placements and under what circumstances. Examples are described in Chapter 7.

Other interventions or services that are commonly needed by elderly victims have been adapted for emergency use and access. Examples include emergency shelter, emergency orders of protection, and temporary guardianships, which are described later.

Ensuring Victim Safety

Among the interventions commonly used to ensure victim safety are safety planning, shelters, and orders of protection.

Safety Planning

Safety planning helps victims consider their situations and decide what to do if they are in danger. It is often used during periods of heightened risk (e.g., after a victim has told someone about the abuse or secured an order of protection) or when victims choose to remain in dangerous situations. Safety planning assumes that victims who have planned for and rehearsed what they will do are more likely to protect themselves when in danger. The process can further help break through denial about what has happened and the seriousness of the abuse.

Safety planning is increasingly being used with elderly victims. Elements included in safety plans depend on the type of risk and its immediacy but generally involve the following:

- Identifying safe contacts. Many elderly victims have never told anyone about the abuse. The first step in safety planning may, therefore, be choosing a family member or friend to confide in. That person may then be asked to check in on the elder, contact someone if the elder is not heard from or cannot be reached, or assist in emergencies.

- Deciding where to go in emergencies; practicing how to leave safely; and developing lists with phone numbers for emergency services including shelters, transportation, and home-care relief workers.
- Packing a bag with clothes, important documents, and money; and leaving it at the home of a family member or friend.
- Devising a code word to use with family or friends in front of the abuser to let them know that the elder needs help.
- Obtaining patients' consent to contact family members, churches, synagogues, and service providers to inform them of concerns.

A primary consideration in safety planning with elderly victims is addressing physical and communication barriers. For example, elders with mobility problems may need mobile phones and special arrangements to leave their homes; or those with impaired vision, hearing, or dexterity may need adapted phones or automatic dialing. "Lifelines," which are portable help buttons for people who are ill or at risk for falls, have also been used. This option, however, requires that elders have "responders" who will check on them when they activate the devices. In addition, safety plans may include support services and orders of protection. Special attention to accessing money or financial documents that are under the abuser's control may also be needed.

Shelters

Elderly victims need shelter for a variety of reasons (Nerenberg, 2002; Wolf, 2001). Some victims may require a safe haven from abusers, whereas others just need a place to stay if they are evicted from homes or apartments, if their homes are unsafe, if caregivers have abandoned them, if caregivers have been fired or arrested, or if essential utilities have been discontinued.

The type of shelter that victims need depends on their functional abilities, their abusers' disposition (are they actively pursuing victims?), the type of abuse, and victims' formal and informal support networks. Some victims may need help on an emergency basis, whereas others need transitional housing as they seek new, permanent homes.

A variety of approaches have been taken to meet elderly victims' need for shelter. These range from helping battered women's shelters accommodate older women to offering victims rooms in long-term care facilities. Although battered women's shelters have historically prioritized younger women with children, they are increasingly serving older women (Vinton, 1998). Some have made special accommodations such as reserving beds or rooms for elders, adapting facilities to make them more accessible, providing training to employees and volunteers in the special needs of older women, and developing special policies such as permitting personal care attendants to visit or stay with residents. However, some professionals and advocates have expressed skepticism about the appropriateness of traditional shelters for older women. But a study by the Older Women's Network in Ontario found that older women were not as concerned as service providers about potential problems (Older Women's Network, n.d.). The study "did not find sufficient reason to establish separate facilities for abused older women." The experiences of one mainstream shelter in working with an elderly guest are described in Chapter 10.

A very different approach is the use of long-term care facilities to provide shelter. In some communities, nursing homes and residential care facilities reserve beds for elderly victims or accept them on a "space available" basis. However, admitting victims on an emergency basis may require that facilities make special arrangements with licensing or monitoring agencies. They may, for example, need to waive requirements for physical examinations prior to admission.

Other options that have been explored include making arrangements with senior housing facilities, hotels, motels, and homeless shelters to accept elderly victims. Eligibility criteria, protocols, resources, services, staffing, and so on vary widely.

The following examples reflect the wide range of shelter options that have been developed around the United States and Canada:

Δ The Dwelling Place Shelter for Abused Elderly in Washington, D.C., is a seven-bed transitional shelter for abused, neglected, or financially exploited seniors. The shelter is operated by So Others Might Eat (SOME, Inc.), an organization that also operates a homeless shelter.

Δ The Harry & Jeanette Weinberg House in New York consists of beds for abused elders that are scattered within New York's Hebrew Home for the Aged.

Δ The Senior Women's Transition House in British Columbia, Canada's first transition house for abused older women, allows residents to stay for up to six months in a four-unit facility. The shelter receives funding from Canada's federal housing agency.

Δ The Maricopa Elder Abuse Prevention Alliance (MEAPA) of Phoenix, Arizona got local residential care facilities and nursing homes to agree to provide free emergency shelter to victims of abuse, neglect, and exploitation. When police or others find victims who need shelter, they bring them to a hospital emergency room to be assessed for medical conditions and eligibility for shelter placement. ER staff then refer eligible patients to on-call MEAPA *volunteers who contact the nearest participating residential care facility with vacancies.*

Δ *The Vermont Network Against Domestic Violence and Sexual Assault established six safe homes across the state. The homes are private residences whose owners or occupants agreed to provide temporary shelter to elderly victims.*

Δ *The Elder Shelter in Omaha, Nebraska, was designed collaboratively by the community's APS unit, police department, and a visiting nurses program. The majority of its clients are victims of neglect.*

Protective Orders

Protective orders are court-issued orders to protect people from harm or harassment. The orders vary across the country but generally fall into two categories: those initiated by prosecutors or judges as part of criminal cases and those initiated by victims in civil actions (Brandl et al., 2007). Criminal orders are usually issued when perpetrators have been arrested.

To file civil restraining orders, victims typically must come to a court, legal clinic, or law office to fill out the paper work. There are several types of orders. Civil harassment orders protect individuals who are being stalked, threatened, or seriously bothered; and domestic violence orders offer protection against abusive family members including intimate partners, sons, and daughters.

Provisions that can typically be requested include the following:

- **Personal conduct orders** prevent restrained parties from abusing, attacking, striking, stalking, threatening, harassing, or contacting the protected party, or destroying their personal property.
- **Stay-away orders** provide that restrained parties must stay a specified distance (e.g., one hundred yards) away from protected persons and their homes, jobs, workplaces, vehicles, and/or other places.
- **Residence exclusions,** or "move-out" orders, require restrained persons to move out of protected persons' residences.
- **No-contact orders** prohibit restrained persons from contacting victims.
- **Other.** Orders may contain a variety of additional provisions such as requiring restrained persons to surrender firearms.

Restraining orders may be available on an emergency or temporary basis. Emergency protective orders (EPOs) are typically issued at the request of law enforcement personnel who have been called to victims' residences (typically for domestic violence). The process is initiated when officers contact the court and speak with judicial officers who order the EPOs over the phone. They then fill out the EPO forms, serve them on the restrained persons (if they can be located), and give copies to protected persons and courts. Temporary orders of protection may be issued by civil courts when cases are first filed and are valid until the next court date is set. If offenders violate orders, the protected parties can call the police or file contempt actions.

> Many of the elder abuse cases that we see involve abuse by a family member, most often an adult child or grandchild. Often, the abusive family member has a substance abuse problem or mental impairment and may be dependent upon the elder for housing or financial needs. The abuser may become verbally abusive toward the elder, yelling and swearing at the elder, and/or calling the elder names. The abuse may escalate to include demands for money, threats, and even physical violence toward the elder. Particularly in situations where the abuser is living with the elder, protective orders play a vital role in separating the parties and thereby ensure the safety of the elder. (Judy Hitchcock, San Francisco's Legal Assistance to the Elderly)

The effectiveness of protective orders in preventing elder abuse is not known, and a number of problems have been reported. For example, elders with physical impairments may find it difficult to come to court, a law office, or a clinic to file papers. Furthermore, domestic violence orders do not apply in many elder abuse cases (e.g., when the abuse is by an unrelated caregiver). And many victims do not want to sever all contact with perpetrators. Finally, victims who have difficulty using the phone may not be able to contact police. Efforts to overcome these obstacles have been initiated by states and courts. For more on what states have done, see Chapter 7. For more on what courts have done, see Chapter 6.

Healing, Empowerment, and Support

The following services can help victims overcome the impact of abuse, gain or regain control over their lives, and reduce the risk of future abuse.

Counseling

Counseling has emerged as one of the most highly valued services available to victims. A Canadian survey of elder abuse victims found that more than 20% would find counseling helpful to them (Podnieks & Pillemer, 1990). When clinicians counsel victims of elder abuse, they draw from various disciplines and models and are likely to focus on the following issues:

- **Coping with crises.** Few people, during times of crisis, have the skills needed to accurately assess their situations and determine what they need to do. For more on crisis counseling, refer to the previous section Crises and Emergencies.
- **Posttrauma stress.** Posttrauma counseling helps victims understand the psychological effects of what has happened to them and develop skills to cope with the situation. It may focus on developing relaxation and coping techniques or gradually decreasing victims' sensitivity to feared objects, people, or situations. Alternatively, it may focus on helping victims examine their thought patterns and learn to combat negative and nonproductive thinking. Group counseling allows people to interact with others and learn that their fears and feelings are not uncommon.
- **Overcoming resistance and denial.** Resistance to treatment or change may stem from fear of retaliation or making matters worse, denial, negative past experiences with service providers, or pessimism (Quinn & Tomita, 1997). As described in Chapter 3, victims may adopt the neutralization techniques used by their abusers to justify, rationalize, or deny abuse. Counselors can sometimes help victims overcome these obstacles by acknowledging and validating their discomfort and ambivalence, empathizing with and accepting their feelings; exploring fears, anxieties, and expectations; providing information; and assigning tasks that are easily accomplished before progressing to larger ones.

One of the earliest approaches to overcoming resistance was the "staircase model" (Breckman & Adelman, 1988), which described three stages that victims go through in getting help: reluctance, recognition, and rebuilding. During the "reluctance stage," victims deny that abuse has occurred, blame themselves, or are ambivalent. They may be unwilling to accept any options, or they may only agree to services that improve their situations without acknowledging abuse, such as home health services or meals-on-wheels. During this stage, caseworkers are encouraged to maintain contact with victims. During the "recognition stage," there is less denial and self-blame. Victims begin to recognize their need for help and may disclose the problem to others even if they are unwilling to accept interventions. During this stage, caseworkers are advised to counsel clients on their options. During the "rebuilding stage" clients no longer blame themselves and are willing to accept help.

Other techniques that may help victims overcome resistance and denial and achieve other goals include:

- **Reality orientation.** Victims are likely to believe that they are responsible for the abuse, that their abusers will change, or that abuse isn't as bad as others make it out to be. They may minimize their own needs, feel that they do not deserve better treatment, or see abusive conduct as normal. Some victims lose confidence in trustworthy individuals or in their ability to judge others' character. Reality orientation helps victims overcome these unrealistic or distorted beliefs, perceptions, and expectations; and make realistic assessments about the abuse, their abusers, and their ability to protect themselves or manage independently. This can be accomplished by providing victims with information or evidence that helps them see situations more realistically. For example, victims who do not believe that trusted persons committed abuse may change their minds when shown compelling evidence of wrongdoing such as forged checks or criminal records. Victims who believe that "the abuse wasn't so bad" can be reminded of its seriousness with pictures of their injuries.
- **Exploring counterproductive relationships with troubled perpetrators.** When older people are abused by mentally ill, substance abusing, or other troubled family members, it can be particularly confusing and painful. Victims may believe they are to blame or that reporting will result in police action that is unfair or cruel. Counselors who work with victims of abuse by troubled family members are increasingly adopting techniques used by groups like the National Alliance for the Mentally Ill (NAMI) and Al Anon. NAMI helps families understand specific illnesses, protect themselves against violence, understand the needs of family members with mental illnesses, and advocate for loved ones in the criminal justice system. Al Anon helps families understand addiction and how it affects them. It further helps families understand their role in "enabling" family members to continue abusing drugs and alcohol. The techniques of "tough love," an approach developed for the parents of troubled teens, which also addresses "enabling behavior," have also been adapted to help families understand that these behaviors do not help.
- **Options counseling.** Counseling helps victims explore their legal rights and service options. Rather than simply referring clients to services, counselors walk clients through the steps they need to take or even rehearse complex procedures.
- **Addressing mental health problems.** Depression, anxiety, isolation, and low self-esteem are all associated with elder abuse. It is not always clear, however, whether these conditions heightened

elders' vulnerability to abuse or if the abuse provoked or contributed to the problems (National Research Council, 2003). In
either case, victims' quality of life can be improved by easing or
eliminating these conditions.

- **Grief counseling and services.** Grief is the response to traumatic
losses such as the loss of loved ones, health, independence, or pos-
sessions. The relationship between elder abuse and traumatic loss
is duel-directional: clinicians have observed that grief and loss
increase elders' vulnerability to abuse, neglect, and exploitation
(Dean Crisp, 2002), and astute predators have long recognized
the vulnerability of grieving elders and used it to their advantage.
On the other hand, abuse may result in traumatic losses, including
the loss of health, independence, homes, life savings, or other pos-
sessions. When elders are betrayed by individuals they loved and
trusted, it can be particularly traumatic (Deem, 2000).

Although grief is a natural response to loss, prolonged and untreated
grief can lead to isolation, depression, self-neglect, somatic or behavioral symptoms, panic disorders, anxiety, post-traumatic stress disorder (PTSD), and substance abuse. Grief counseling may be performed
by social workers, nurses, psychologists, marriage and family therapists,
medical professionals, and clergy. Individual or group counseling may be
indicated at any point during the grief process. Grief counseling may even
begin before an impending death.

When working with victims of elder abuse, grief counselors need to
address victims' heightened vulnerability. Counselors need to understand,
for example, how predators play upon grief to exploit elders and learn
skills to help elders withstand undue influence. They also need to recognize that the death of a spouse or caregiver may leave elders without care
or place them in the position of managing their own finances for the first
time. The elders may therefore need support services, new social networks,
and new skills such as managing finances or finding others to help.

- **Substance abuse counseling and treatment.** Although substance
abuse by either the abuser or the victim has frequently been
cited as a risk factor for elder abuse, few service programs have
addressed it. Bradshaw and Spencer (1999) attribute this failure
to "a pervasive view among service providers that substance abusers can't be helped or that in doing so, practitioners are, in effect,
'enabling' the person with the problem."

Like other mental health problems associated with elder abuse and
neglect, substance abuse may heighten elders' vulnerability to abuse, or

it may be a response to it. In either case, treatment can improve seniors' quality of life.

Traditional treatment for substance abuse is provided in hospitals, therapeutic communities, or outpatient programs, and generally begins with detoxification in controlled settings. Medications may be used to control drug cravings and relieve severe symptoms of withdrawal. For most patients, a combination of medication and individual or group therapy is most effective. Traditional counseling approaches help people understand their behavior and motivations, develop higher self-esteem, cope with stress, and gain insight into how alcohol and drugs have affected their lives and those of others. Self-help groups provide support and reinforce messages learned in treatment. Traditional substance abuse programs also assume that persons must be motivated to engage in the treatment process. For some, that may mean "hitting bottom" before they are ready to accept help. Traditional programs also typically require total abstinence. Perhaps the most widely recognized program is Alcoholics Anonymous (AA), which offers free, peer-led support groups.

Some experts question the appropriateness of traditional substance abuse prevention programs for elders, pointing out that physical, cognitive, and communication barriers may be an obstacle. Charmaine Spencer, an adjunct professor and research associate at the Gerontology Research Centre, Simon Fraser University in Vancouver, British Columbia, notes, "For seniors, hitting bottom can mean death. Or, it may mean becoming so incapacitated that they're institutionalized. And the 'helping hand' may not be there for them" (Nerenberg, 2000). Spencer and her colleagues suggest that "harm reduction," may be a more appropriate approach for elders. Harm reduction is a nonjudgmental, nonconfrontational, and noncoercive approach. It addresses drug use as a complex and multifaceted problem, which may be related to isolation, past trauma, poverty, and discrimination (Bradshaw & Spencer, 1999). The approach recognizes that although alcohol or drugs are harmful to elders, other harms may be more serious at certain points. It calls for practitioners to adopt a nonjudgmental attitude, work at clients' pace, and not insist on abstinence, but instead, deal with immediate threats.

Few counseling programs specifically target victims of elder abuse. One, "The Elder Abuse Therapy Program" at San Francisco's Institute on Aging (IOA), is housed within the agency's geriatric psychology training program.[4] Every student in the program receives training in elder abuse prevention. Counseling is psychodynamic and client centered, which means, according to the program's supervisor, Melissa Anderson:

We take our cues from clients and wait for things to unfold. I pay attention to how people relate to me and how I feel about them, which tells me a lot about how they relate to other people. That feedback can be important. For some, consistently having someone come to their homes and listening to them for an hour is important in itself. It conveys a sense of entitlement and the message that they have a right to be safe.

Support Groups

Support groups, which have been adapted from the fields of domestic violence and caregiving, have begun to feature prominently in elder abuse practice. The term "support group" traditionally referred to informal gatherings of people who were experiencing similar life events and were led by laypersons. The assumption behind groups is that people who have had similar experiences are better equipped than family, friends, or professionals to understand and empathize and that the mutual exchange of information between members is a powerful experience that can induce lasting change. Groups further help members learn new ways to handle challenges, cope with change, maintain new behaviors, and build social networks. In recent years, the term has also been applied to more formal groups led by professionals using therapeutic and educational methods.

The Milwaukee Women's Center (MWC) launched one of the nation's first support groups for older battered women in 1991. The groups, patterned after groups for younger women, were a component of a broader program that also included case management, shelter, and counseling. Topics of discussion included power and control, the dynamics of family violence, and safety planning (Seaver, 1996).

> You have to understand the isolation and shame of living with abuse. There are all kinds of reasons why victims can't talk about their abuse. But when the women come to the support group, they can actually talk about it, laugh, and cry. It's a real relief. (Carole Seaver, 1995)

Other communities followed suit. A 1997 survey revealed thirty support groups for elderly victims of abuse in the United States and Canada. Of these, there was an almost even division of groups operated by domestic violence programs and those operated by aging service programs (sixteen and fourteen respectively) (Wolf, 2001). Another survey commissioned by AARP a few years later identified thirty-four groups and described their key features (Brandl, Hebert, Rozwadowski, & Spangler, 2003). Although most group participants were women who had been abused by spouses or intimate partners, some groups included both men and women participants who had been abused by intimate partners and other family members (Brandl et al., 2003). At least one program offered separate groups for victims abused by intimate partners and those abused by children, and a few groups were culturally specific.

These early surveys yielded recommendations for other organizations that were interested in starting support groups. Respondents highlighted the importance of using leaders or coleaders who are elderly themselves or familiar with aging issues, and pointed out the need for extensive outreach. They further noted that, for some participants, transportation was a problem. They also emphasized the importance of collaboration among domestic violence coalitions, state units on aging, adult protective services, and victim assistance programs.

Podnieks (1999) has called for the expanded use of support groups and notes their potential benefits for members of diverse cultural communities. She further points out their potential benefits for others, besides victims, including caregivers, employees of long-term care facilities, and even the grandchildren of victims. She also offers recommendations for organizing and facilitating groups.

The lines between support groups and therapy groups may be gray. Melissa Anderson of the Institute on Aging in San Francisco, which also offers groups, had this to say about how groups function and evolve over time:

> Each group is different. At one point, ours was mostly "psycho-educational." The members wanted speakers. Later, group members started using their relationships with each other more and it became a more serious support group. When an older psychotherapist became the leader, there was a palpable shift.
>
> We get a lot of parents who are abused by adult children with mental illnesses. At one point, four out of six group members had children with bi-polar disorder. In some cases it's not the abuser with the mental illness, but other family members. We also see what I call "spousal abuse by proxy," women whose abusive husbands are dead and whose sons now abuse them.
>
> There's a lot of discussion about safety plans. Recently, when a member's son was released from a locked psychiatric facility into a board and care home, he went AWOL and she was terrified. But she had her bag packed, and a friend helped her take the subway to stay with a daughter. There's also a lot of discussion about members' frustration with agencies. They think agencies aren't doing enough to help them. It's hard for clients to know how they're playing into that, which we talk about.
>
> Building social networks is another goal, and some members talk to each other between meetings or check up on members who miss sessions. Interestingly, I think the group has helped some members

understand how to use other people in their lives for support. One member came to group one day and said, "Before, I would never have talked to anyone at my church about this. Now, I look around and I say, 'Aha, I could trust *her*!'"

Little is known about the impact of support groups, and what is known is based largely on anecdotal evidence and small surveys that measure clients' and providers' satisfaction (Podnieks, 1999). Participants generally evaluate support groups favorably and credit the groups with helping them develop mutual support relationships with peers, move beyond guilt, enhance self-esteem, learn problem-solving and coping strategies, and develop survival strategies. Studies, in fact, have found that support groups are among the few services that victims believe are helpful and would be willing to accept (Brownell, Berman, & Salamone, 1999; Podnieks, 1999).

One support group evaluation explored the impact of a "psycho-educational support group" that met for two hours a week for ten weeks (Brownell & Heiser, 2006). The survey measured changes in members' risk, depression, guilt, anxiety, health, self-esteem, and their sense of social support. Although the study failed to substantiate changes in any of these areas, the researchers observed that study participants did "appear to demonstrate a readiness to move to another level of intervention: that of recognizing their own level of expertise in elder abuse and developing the skills to become peer counselors and assume the role of leaders in the elder abuse movement."

Preserving, Protecting, and Recovering Assets

Protecting, preserving, and recovering victims' assets are among the greatest challenges in serving financial abuse victims. Clearly, the most effective approach is to prevent financial abuse from occurring in the first place. This can be accomplished by safeguarding vulnerable elders' assets through daily money management, ensuring that advance directives such as powers of attorney and trusts are crafted to offer maximum protection, and helping vulnerable elders withstand the advances of financial predators.

Daily Money Management

Elders who are unable to manage their money as a result of cognitive or physical impairments are particularly vulnerable to exploitation resulting from the misuse of legal documents, fraud, coercion, trickery, or undue influence. These elders may be preyed upon by family members, acquaintances, employees, or predators (Nerenberg, 2003). Elders who lack experience managing money may also be at heightened risk. This includes elders who assume responsibility for money management after the death of a spouse and recent immigrants from countries with "cash economies," who are unfamiliar with banking practices (Wilber & Cedano, 2002). Daily money management (DMM) can help prevent financial loss to vulnerable elders. In can further reduce vulnerability to other forms of abuse, such as violence, neglect, or intimidation, when financial gain is the motive.

DMM is provided by public agencies; private, nonprofit agencies; and for-profit businesses, including banks, and is tailored to meet clients' specific needs. People with moderate memory loss, for example, may still be able to make decisions about their money but may require help writing and signing checks, balancing checkbooks, budgeting, managing credit, and other tasks (Wilber, 1995). These clients generally retain control over their assets.

When clients are unable to make reasonable decisions about their finances or consent to transactions, money managers may need legal authority to do so for them. The manager may request that the Social Security Administration, the Department of Veterans Affairs, or other providers of government benefits appoint them as "representative payees" (also called "substitute payees"), which gives them authority to manage government payments. Other options include powers of attorney for finances and trusts, which can only be executed before the onset of incapacity when elders fully understand the documents.

Specific steps that daily money managers can take to reduce the risk of abuse include the following:

- Monitoring bank statements and other financial documents
- Paying bills and ensuring that rent, debts, or other revenues owed to elders are collected
- Requesting and reviewing receipts from home-care workers
- Arranging for automatic deposits of pension, public benefit, and other checks so that they do not come to elders' homes where they can be accessed by perpetrators
- Removing seniors' contact information from marketers' lists and reporting infractions to appropriate law enforcement or regulatory agencies
- Checking elders' credit reports for debt incurred by others
- Require third parties to sign checks or contracts, withdraw funds, authorize payments, and so on

There has been little research to explore the effectiveness of DMM in maximizing independence or reducing the risk of abuse. A notable exception is a study that examined the use of DMM as a less restrictive alternative to guardianship. The study found that DMM enhanced financial security and reduced financial exploitation (Wilber, 1995). Another unpublished evaluation of a model project in Southern California also affirmed the effectiveness of DMM in preventing financial abuse and went further in outlining the characteristics of clients who use the service (Wilber & Cedano, 2002). According to the study, those most likely to use DMM are elders with impaired executive control function. As a result of DMM, these clients were less likely to experience fraud and financial exploitation, and more likely to pay their bills on time. Program personnel were also successful in securing more entitlement money for participants. Client satisfaction with the program was high, and most clients reported that they had close and trusting relationships with their financial assistants and that the service had increased their independence (Wilber & Cedano, 2002).

Fraud Prevention Programs

Fraud prevention programs alert seniors to scams and provide them with the skills and strategies they need to avoid exploitation. Many advocates have begun to acknowledge the need to go beyond simple "scam alerts" to help elders identify fraudulent sales tactics, resist aggressive advances, and report fraudulent telemarketers and door-to-door solicitors to law enforcement (Aziz, Bolick, Kleinman, & Shadel, 2000). Following are some examples of successful fraud prevention programs:

Δ *The National Telemarketing Victim Call Center is operated by WISE Senior Services in Los Angeles in collaboration with the FBI, U.S. Postal Inspectors, and a telephone company. The program uses volunteers to staff a "reverse boiler room." The term boiler room refers to an office that is used by fraudulent telemarketers. The high-pressure techniques they use to pitch the scams account for the name. Scammers typically use "sucker" or "mooch" lists, which contain contact information for people who have been victimized in the past. Similarly, the Call Center volunteers use lists that have been confiscated by law enforcement agencies. They call the elders on these lists and warn them that they have been targeted (Aziz, Bolick, Kleinman, & Shadel, 2000). A program in Oregon uses a similar approach but added a friendly visitor component. Elders who are believed to be particularly vulnerable are offered the opportunity to talk to volunteers who have received special training in fraud prevention.*

Δ *"Striking Back: Elder Financial Abuse Prevention" was designed by educators from Florida and Tennessee to teach elders how* to deal with telemarketers and door-to-door solicitors (Guion, Turner, & Wise, 2004). Launched in 2002, the program draws from research findings that suggest that older adults have trouble hanging up on telemarketers, and that the length of time they spend on the phone increases their risk. Elderly participants are provided with educational materials, which include practice scenarios based on actual cases involving telemarketing schemes and door-to-door solicitors. Working in pairs, they identify specific schemes and techniques, develop responses to common pitches, determine what harm the scheme can cause, and discuss what information is being solicited and how it can be used to further defraud victims. The program provides participants with thirteen strategies for refusing solicitations that range from hanging up the phone or closing the door, to telling callers that someone else manages their financial affairs.

In order to evaluate the program's impact and determine what strategies elderly participants favored, the researchers made mock telemarketing calls to participants. The results were promising, with half of the participants using at least one of the thirteen strategies. The greatest percentage of participants (26%) ended calls by saying "Sorry, I am not interested" followed by "I'm too (ill, busy, annoyed, cranky, distracted) to talk now" (20%). Participants rejected strategies that relinquished their independent decision making (e.g., "Someone else handles my finances") and strategies that suggested they did not trust callers.

Δ A project to prevent identity theft in nursing homes was initiated by the Michigan attorney general's office. The project was begun in response to the discovery that nursing home employees, temp workers, and people posing as employees were using their positions to get information about residents and using it to commit identity (ID) theft. Under project "It's MI Identity," investigators track ID theft in nursing homes statewide and conduct routine credit checks for all nursing home residents.[5]

Δ The Fair Lending Project for Seniors of the Council on Aging Silicon Valley protects seniors from "predatory lending," a practice in which mortgage brokers and loan officers target homebuyers and homeowners for "subprime" purchase and refinance loans. Sub-prime loans are typically made to people who do not qualify for standard loans because of low credit scores and histories of payment delinquencies, charge-offs, or bankruptcies. Although not all victims are elderly, seniors are three times more likely to be offered sub-prime loans than similarly situated younger people regardless of their credit worthiness (Walters & Hermanson, 2001).

*The Fair Lending Project, in partnership with the Fair Hous-
ing Law Project and several other legal and social service providers, conducts community education and outreach events. Project
staff also "universally screen" potential victims. Universal screening is when all the seniors at a partner site or event are asked
about their experiences with home loans. There are two types of
universal screening tools. One is a questionnaire that is distributed at outreach presentations, which seniors fill out themselves
and the other is a set of questions that staff at partner sites fill
out for elders during face to face interviews. Universal screening is based on the assumption that seniors may not volunteer
information about problems but will respond to direct questions.
The technique also serves to raise awareness about the problem.
Fair Lending Project staff review the screening tools and contact
seniors who indicate that they have problems that require follow
up. Free social work and legal services are provided.*

*According to Shawna Reeves Nourzaie, a social worker with
the project:*

> I would say that the top five problems with our clients' lend-
> ing experiences are (1) falsified income and bogus appraisals
> resulting in high loan amounts with unaffordable monthly
> payments, (2) prepayment penalties that make it hard if not
> impossible to refinance into better loans, (3) undisclosed inter-
> est rates and hidden fees, (4) broker abuses including bait and
> switch tactics, lies, and pressure, (5) loan disclosure docu-
> ments that are not in the borrower's language. Adding insult
> to injury, our clients with these bad loans usually have terrific
> credit, meaning they could have qualified for loans with much
> better terms.

Reducing the Risk of Financial Abuse Involving Powers of Attorney

It has frequently been observed that many of the instruments that were
created to assist and protect people with disabilities can become "licenses
to steal" when they end up in the wrong hands. Virtually any financial
or legal instrument can be used to exploit, including powers of attorney, trusts, guardianships, reverse mortgages, annuities, home equity
loans, and quitclaim deeds. Marriage and adoptions can also be tactics
of exploitation. Although it is beyond the scope of this book to describe
what can be done in every situation, abuse involving powers of attorney
is described because of the frequency with which it occurs.

A power of attorney (POA) is a document with which one person
(the principal) grants authority to another (the "agent," or "attorney

in fact") to act on the principal's behalf with regard to the principal's property, personal care, or health care. Powers of attorney for finances give agents the power to manage, dispose of, or sell principals' property, to use the property as security, or to borrow money on the principals' behalf. They may be *limited* or *general*. Limited powers are for specific acts, such as authority to cash checks, whereas general powers grant authority to handle all of the principals' financial affairs. POAs are a useful tool for people who are unable to transact business on their own as a result of disabilities.

Principals must have legal decision-making capacity at the time they execute the powers. "Durable" or "enduring" powers of attorney (DPA) remain in effect beyond the onset of incapacity. Executing DPAs allow competent elders to choose trustworthy people to handle their affairs and continue to do so even if they become incapacitated. The powers may become effective at the time they are signed or, in the case of "springing powers of attorney," at a specified time or event in the future (e.g., the DPA will "spring"—become valid—only if and when the principal becomes incapacitated). Traditionally, POAs have terminated if principals lost capacity unless the POAs contained language stating that they were intended to be durable (i.e., "This power of attorney shall not be affected by the subsequent incapacity of the principal."). In 2006, however, the National Conference of Commissioners on Uniform State Laws (NCCUSL)[6] revised its Uniform Durable Power of Attorney to make it durable (survive incapacity) unless expressly indicated otherwise. It may be anticipated that many states will adopt this approach. For more information on the uniform durable power of attorney and actions states have taken to reduce abuse of powers of attorney, see Chapter 7.

Powers of attorney, when granted to responsible parties, can prevent abuse by ensuring that elders' property and assets are supervised and inaccessible to those who seek to exploit. They are fairly simple and inexpensive to create and can eliminate the need for guardianship. POAs are a good idea for people who have others they can completely trust.

There is, however, little oversight of POAs, and the following abuses are common:

- Principals are coerced into signing.
- Principals who lack mental capacity sign them (the principal must understand the document at the time of signing regardless of the type of POA).
- The agent uses the power after it has terminated (the principal has become incapacitated and the power is not a durable one).
- The agent uses the POA for purposes other than those for which it was intended.

- Agents transfer principals' property to themselves without authorization.
- Agents do not act solely in the interest of principals.

Professionals are increasingly encouraging seniors and their families to consult with trusted advisers and attorneys when drafting POAs to ensure that they are as "theft-proof" as possible. Attorney Ellen Henningsen (2000) advises attorneys to (1) clearly explain the limits of the agent's authority; (2) include documentation affirming that agents are aware of the limits to their authority; (3) educate agents about their financial responsibilities and limitations; and (4) include "oversight" provisions.

Preserving and Recovering Assets

The likelihood of victims recovering stolen assets or property or being compensated for them is very slim because perpetrators are likely to hide assets (both those of their victims and their own). When financial abuse investigations are in progress, perpetrators are likely to move quickly to drain bank accounts or expedite financial transactions. This makes it critical that responders also move quickly to secure and preserve assets that are in jeopardy. This can be accomplished through both informal means and legal interventions. Informal means include contacting banks or financial institutions to inform them that APS or law enforcement agencies are investigating abuse involving their customers and asking for their voluntary cooperation. This may include "red flagging" accounts or postponing transactions.

Some states, local communities, and other organizations have developed formal means for "freezing" or "seizing" assets or stopping transactions. Some of these formal means include the following:

- In California, specially trained peace officers can issue declarations to public guardians when there is cause to believe that crimes are being committed against incapacitated persons and they are in danger of losing their property (California Probate Code §2952). The declarations must be cosigned by supervisors of local APS units and presented to public guardians who can take immediate possession or control of the property stated in the declaration. The Santa Clara Rapid Response Financial Abuse Specialist Team, which is described in Chapter 6, frequently uses this intervention and others to quickly preserve assets.
- As part of a pilot project in Pennsylvania, one county hired a retired FBI agent and another county hired an accountant/

insurance fraud investigator to work with APS on financial abuse cases to focus on asset recovery. These "asset investigators," who "follow the money" while investigations are in progress, are credited with recovering millions of dollars and multiple prosecutions (National Center on Elder Abuse, 2003).

- The U.S. attorney's office in San Francisco employed a special "asset investigator" as part of a pilot project to increase the recovery rates of court-ordered restitution and fines (Nerenberg, 1999). The investigator worked alongside probation officials and U.S. attorneys who were investigating investment and telemarketing fraud.

A variety of legal interventions are also available to protect and recover assets, some of which are described in the next section.

Ensuring Justice

The Civil Justice System

The civil justice system is assuming an increasingly prominent role in elder abuse prevention. Civil law encompasses a broad range of legal matters. Civil lawsuits address conflicts, disagreements, and disputes between individuals, businesses, or organizations. Civil courts also handle "protective proceedings," including guardianships and restraining orders.

Civil Lawsuits. Victims of elder abuse and neglect or their advocates may initiate civil lawsuits against abusers to resolve conflicts or compensate victims for losses, pain, or suffering. The parties instituting the suits, called *plaintiffs*, are the individuals who have been injured, and the offenders are held accountable to them. Unlike criminal courts, which attempt to determine offenders' guilt or innocence, civil courts attempt to determine whether an offender or a third party is legally responsible (civilly liable) for injuries or harm. Findings of liability are rendered by judges or juries or through settlements by the parties. Defendants who are found liable pay monetary damages to victims and/or their families.

There are two primary types of civil cases: "tort claims" and "contract actions."

Tort Claims. Tort claims compensate parties who have been intentionally or negligently hurt or injured, or who suffered from property loss or damage through acts or omissions, malpractice, defamation, and so on. In recent years, a greater number of elder abuse victims have initiated civil tort actions in federal, state, or tribal courts. They initiated these actions to gain compensation for injuries sustained from assaults, negligent care, and the taking of money or property. Some of the common tort actions that are potentially available to victims of elder abuse include the following:

Tort Actions Related to Financial Abuse

- Breach of fiduciary duty. Abuse may be committed by persons who have a fiduciary responsibility or duty toward others, including "attorneys-in-fact," guardians, and trustees. Breaches of fiduciary duty that are common in elder abuse cases include actions that result in financial injury or loss, and using an elder's funds or property for the benefit of the fiduciary.
- **Conversion,** the civil equivalent of theft, is when a person assumes control over the property of another with intent to deprive him or her of the property.
- **Fraud** is an intentional misrepresentation of facts made to deceive someone, which results in harm. Fraud includes telephone, sweepstakes, and home improvement scams. Fraud has also been used as a cause of action when agents have used powers of attorney to abuse principals (Hughes, 2000).
- **Unjust enrichment** occurs when a person benefits unjustly at the expense of another.
- **Tortious interference** is causing harm by disrupting or interfering with a contractual relationship (e.g., interfering with an expected inheritance).

Tort Actions for Harm to Person

- **Assault** is the willful attempt or threat to inflict injury, including displays of force that cause people to fear or expect immediate bodily harm.
- **Battery** is intentional and nonconsensual contact with another person that causes bodily injury or is offensive.
- **Wrongful death** is death caused by another person without justification or excuse.
- **False imprisonment** is holding people against their will or preventing them from moving about freely. It can include the use of physical restraints, removal of an elder's means of transportation (e.g., cane or wheelchair), or locking the elder in a room.
- **Negligence** is the failure to use the care that a reasonably prudent person would use under similar circumstances. For negligence to occur, this failure of care must result in harm. Examples include failure to provide food or shelter or to administer medication in a timely manner.

Contract Actions. The term *contract actions* refers to breaches of duties between individual parties in which plaintiffs claim that defendants broke written, oral, or implied promises. Contract actions may relate to the transfer of money or property, the provision of services, rental agreements, terms of employment, marriage, and other such matters. Contract law provides various remedies to repair the damage and "make injured parties whole." A common form of elder financial exploitation involves abusers who convince elders who lack decision-making capacity to enter into contractual relationships that are extremely favorable to the abusers. In these situations, actions alleging that the elder lacked mental capacity to enter into the contract may be used.

Addressing Abuse in Long-Term Care Facilities. A variety of causes of action have been filed against long-term care facilities, the most common of which is probably negligence (Moskowitz, 2003). These suits may involve allegations of inadequate care, failure to supervise and protect patients from harm, and failure to provide adequate training to, and supervision of, staff. Civil actions for assault and battery have been filed when residents are assaulted by employees or other residents. Lawsuits have also been brought on behalf of residents for unlawful, unfair, fraudulent, or deceptive acts or business practices, unfair methods of competition, or misleading advertising. In addition, state attorneys general have brought civil actions seeking civil penalties and restitution to the Medicaid program for failure to provide adequate care, treatment, and services. Courts may further order improvements to protect current and future residents by raising the level of care, treatment and services.

Other Civil Remedies. Other civil remedies used in elder abuse cases include divorce, separation, and annulment when abuse is by spouses; and constructive trusts, which are involuntary trusts created by courts to benefit parties that have been wrongfully deprived of assets or property through misconduct such as fraud, duress, or abuse of confidential relationships. For example, if someone convinces an elder to deed his or her home to him or her without payment, and the elder sues the person, the court can impose a constructive trust on the property. This means that the defendant no longer owns the property; it is held in trust by the court for the benefit of the elder.

Eviction may be needed when abusers, including family members, live in elders' homes and refuse to leave or pay rent. The methods used to evict someone vary and depend on factors like how an abuser first came into the home and whether rent was ever paid or expected. It may be possible and necessary to evict individuals even when there is no formal lease agreement.

Guardianship. Civil law provides for the appointment of guardians[7] to act on behalf of people who have physical or mental impairments that render them incapable of providing for their basic needs. Most guardians are family members or friends. Private, professional guardians are available in most communities for people who lack family members and friends who are willing or able to serve. Some nonprofit agencies also serve as guardians. And finally, public guardians are public entities that serve as guardians. They are considered by some to be the "guardian of last resort" for people who do not have family members available, and who cannot afford to hire private professionals.

There are two types of guardians: "guardians of estate (or property)" and "guardians of person." Guardians of estate manage financial affairs. They may be appointed when elders are unable to manage their own finances and have been, or are at risk of being, financially abused or unduly influenced. Guardians of person are for people who are unable to provide for their own basic needs such as the need for shelter and food. Guardians of person make decisions about medical treatment, housing, transportation, food preparation, attendant care, and other personal needs.

Guardianship may be used to stop or prevent elder abuse in the following situations (Quinn, 2005):

- When severely impaired victims are unable to grasp the severity of their situation and refuse needed services
- When family members quarrel over the custody or assets of an impaired elder
- When adult children want to claim inheritances prematurely or influence their older family members to make new wills
- When less restrictive legal devises, such as durable powers of attorney or trusts, have been misused.

Specific actions that guardians of estate can take to stop abuse include removing wards' assets from wrongdoers' control (e.g., revoking powers of attorney that have been used to exploit), initiating lawsuits to recover misappropriated assets or property, evicting wrongdoers from elders' residences, selling unneeded property, and purchasing needed services. Guardians of person can authorize medical treatment, arrange for elders to live in safe places, fire abusive attendants, and so on.

Although guardianship is typically involuntary, Eileen Goldman, a consultant to private fiduciaries and nonprofit agencies, provided the following case example of a voluntary guardianship:

> I'm working with a delightful, ninety-seven-year-old man, Sheldon, whose wife of sixty-five years died three years ago. At the time, the

couple was living in a one-bedroom apartment even though a lifetime of hard work and saving had made them multimillionaires.

Soon after Sheldon's wife died, the vultures started circling. His long-term accountant, whom he'd helped out financially for years, started pressuring him for more money. A nephew moved in and started making expensive phone calls. He started pressuring Sheldon to invest in a risky business venture. Sheldon agreed because he was too good-natured to say no. When Sheldon's attorney realized that Sheldon was being pressured and had developed mild dementia, he suggested a private professional guardian. We explained to Sheldon what guardianship was, and he agreed to it.

Now, when Sheldon's friends ask for money, he tells them they have to contact me. When they tell me "He wants to buy me this or that," I tell them I'll get back to them and ask Sheldon in private what he really wants. If he seems unsure, I'll ask him several times during our visits or ask in different ways. If I'm unsure what to do, I ask for an ex parte hearing for instructions. Recently, Sheldon's friends told me that Sheldon wanted to throw a big party at an expensive restaurant for his 98th birthday. When I talked to him in private, he said he'd prefer to just take a few friends out to a restaurant, which I arranged. Voluntary guardianships are unusual, but they happen.

The Criminal Justice System

The criminal justice system handles violations of criminal law. The "plaintiff" in criminal cases is the "people," which refers to the fact that criminal acts are considered to be acts against society. In criminal matters, it is society to whom offenders must answer. The primary goals of the criminal justice system are to determine offenders' guilt or innocence and to make the guilty pay a debt to society through incarceration, probation, or restitution. The benefits and advantages of the criminal justice system for preventing elder abuse were described in Chapter 1.

The criminal justice system operates at the local, state, federal, and tribal levels. Most elder abuse matters are state crimes and are handled by local law enforcement agencies, which include police and sheriffs. Criminal conduct occurring in long-term care facilities is likely to be investigated by Medicaid Fraud Control Units, which are located in offices of state attorneys general. Federal law enforcement agencies investigate certain elder abuse matters that occur in more than one state, some crimes that are committed on Indian reservations and military bases, and federal crimes, which include telemarketing, identity theft, and the like. In addition, federal regulatory agencies have law enforcement branches that investigate and prosecute crimes associated with their specific functions. For example, when frauds and scams are committed through the

mail, the United States Postal Service may investigate. Crimes involving
Indians may be handled by tribal law enforcement agencies, although
a variety of factors affect jurisdiction, including the type and severity of crimes, whether perpetrators and victims are Indian, whether
the crimes occurred on reservations, tribes' legal resources, and other
factors (Jones, 2000).

Depending on the jurisdictions, prosecutors, who represent "the people" in criminal cases, may be district attorneys, attorneys general, or U.S.
attorneys. Many forms of elder abuse correspond to "traditional" crimes
like assault, battery, domestic violence, attempted murder, theft, larceny,
or extortion. Some states, however, have created special offenses that
reflect the special relationships victims are likely to have with their abusers, their heightened vulnerability, the greater impact crimes are likely to
have on them, and the obstacles they are likely to face in seeking justice.

The role of law enforcement personnel in elder abuse is not, however, limited to criminal investigations. In accordance with state law, law
enforcement agencies may do the following:

- Check on the "well-being" of seniors when family members, professionals, or others have concerns but are unable to gain access
- Provide back-up to health and social service providers when they
  respond to reports in potentially dangerous or explosive abuse
  situations
- Secure, serve, or enforce protective orders
- Assist with protective placements of people with mental illnesses who
  pose a danger to themselves and others or who are gravely disabled
- Accept and file reports of abuse, which can be used to establish a
  history of abuse
- Follow through with court-ordered forcible entry and eviction of
  abusers
- Provide background information about known or suspected perpetrators to health and social service providers who are charged
  with responding to abuse reports
- Assist in locating victims and/or perpetrators who cannot be found
- Refer victims, vulnerable and self-neglecting elders, and abusers
  to social service organizations
- Report abuse and neglect discovered during criminal investigations to social service agencies

Mediation

Mediation is the bringing together of parties in disputes, with a neutral
third party, to negotiate agreements, resolve conflicts, or reach consensus.

It may be used as an alternative to the legal system, or courts may advise parties in lawsuits to consider mediation or order them into mediation.

In victim-offender mediation, victims meet offenders in a safe, structured setting and engage in discussions. As described in Chapter 3, victims may tell offenders about the crimes' physical, emotional, and financial impact and ask offenders questions. Victims may also become involved in developing restitution plans.

Chapter 3 also pointed out that many advocates have argued against the use of offender-victim mediation in domestic violence cases. They claim that imbalances in economic, physical, and societal power make it impossible for victims to negotiate on an equal footing with their abusers and may be dangerous because there is no mechanism for holding abusers accountable. Additionally, victims who have suffered from serious physical and sexual assaults may be too traumatized initially to take part in mediation. Some domestic violence advocates suggest that mediation can be used in certain domestic violence situations such as after sentencing, when offenders are in custody.

The Center for Social Gerontology (TCSG) has pioneered the use of mediation as an alternative to guardianship when caregivers who share responsibility for elders are in conflict or having trouble making decisions. TCSG has developed educational materials to help families and professionals understand when and how mediation can be used and has conducted a pilot project in other states.[8] The Georgia Division of Aging Services, Atlanta Department of Human Resources, has also explored the use of mediation to resolve caregiving issues and disputes, avoid premature institutionalization, and preserve families.[9]

Mediation has also been used to resolve financial abuse cases. The following case serves as an example:

> Roger, a man in his late forties with a developmental disability, was living with his grandmother, Cecelia, in Cecelia's extremely deteriorated home. Roger had moved in with Cecelia years earlier after his mother died. At that time, Roger had inherited a house from his mother. An uncle, Luke, who managed Roger's finances, sold the house and used the proceeds to purchase a vacation home, promising to send Roger monthly payments, which he never did. When Cecelia developed dementia, Luke became her representative payee, but he failed to pay her the full monthly payments.
>
> Roger was referred to a private, nonprofit guardianship program, which became his guardian of estate, and another guardian was found for Cecelia. Because Cecelia required more care than Roger could provide but lacked the funds to pay for in-home care, her guardian explored reverse annuity mortgages to cover the costs. However, the lenders were only willing to give her a $100,000 loan, which would have only lasted a couple of years. After this time, the home would

have to be sold to repay the loan and Cecelia and Roger would have to find a new home. In reviewing her documents, it was discovered that Cecelia had executed a will leaving her home to Luke. Because she no longer had capacity, she could not change the will.

Roger's guardian hired an attorney, who filed a lawsuit against Luke on Roger's behalf for fraud and elder and dependent adult abuse. As Roger's lawsuit progressed, the Court referred the parties to mediation to see if an agreement could be reached to resolve the issues. The mediation resulted in a settlement agreement whereby Luke agreed to give up his future interest in Cecelia's home and to make monthly payments to Cecelia to cover her care needs up to a maximum of $240,000. In exchange for these payments, Cecilia's guardian sought and received court permission to transfer title to Cecelia's home to Roger.

According to Nancy Rasch, the attorney in the case, "What made this an interesting mediation is that we were able to consider the intertwined needs of both Cecilia and Roger, rather than focusing solely on a remedy for Roger. In a typical settlement, Luke would pay damages to Roger, and we would not have been able to address Cecelia's needs. The way it turned out, Roger got a home to make up for the one he'd never been paid for, Cecelia got the care she needed, the two were able to continue living together, which is what they wanted, and Luke was held accountable.

"I always consider mediation in financial abuse cases because it gives you more flexibility than litigation. It also gives clients a chance to hear the other side. Often, lawyers tell clients, 'You have a great case,' which may be a great case from their perspective but not from the clients'. Mediation gives them a chance to hear the other parties' side without the lawyer's 'filter.'"

Conferencing (or Family Group Conferencing)

As described in Chapter 3, conferencing is one of several techniques associated with "restorative justice." Conferences provide an opportunity for people who are directly and indirectly affected by conflicts to express support for victims and offenders, agree on offenders' responsibilities, consider alternatives, and negotiate outcomes. Participants include victims' and perpetrators' families, friends, supporters, health and social service providers, spiritual advisers, and key community members. Following are two examples of programs that use conferencing:

Δ *The Jamestown S'Klallam Family Group Conferencing Project was a three-year research and demonstration project sponsored by the Administration on Aging as part of the Native American Caregiver Support Program. It explored the use of conferences to help families that are in conflict or having difficulties related to caregiving, including burnout and sibling rivalry, the need to address end-of-life issues, and confronting anger and guilt (Nerenberg, Baldridge, & Benson, 2003).*

Δ *The Community Care Access Centre's Restorative Justice Approaches to Elder Abuse (Waterloo, Ontario) uses "talking circles" in elder abuse cases to restore relationships (Groh, 2003). Concerned parties meet to explore why the abuse occurred, what can be done to repair the harm, and what can be done to prevent it from happening again. The project was designed in recognition of the fact that many seniors fail to report abuse or seek outside help for fear of losing their relationships with abusive family members or friends. The program is being replicated in other cities.*

One situation that was referred to our program was an elderly woman who was being cared for by her brother. Culturally, he perceived it as his obligation to provide care, but as he aged, this became difficult. One day, in frustration, he struck her. He was charged with assault, and the Crown agreed to diversion. Eventually, with adequate preparation, the people affected by the abuse came together in a circle process. The "accused" was extremely apologetic. He recognized that he was no longer able to care for his sister. The sister understood and accepted this apology. The family identified that they had an obligation to help, reached consensus about how to do so, and developed a care plan. The charges were dropped, and everyone expressed satisfaction with the process and outcome. (Arlene Groh, Project Coordinator, Community Care Access Centre of Waterloo)

INTERVENTIONS FOR PERPETRATORS AND THOSE AT RISK FOR ABUSING

As described in Chapter 1, in recent years, the field of elder abuse prevention has directed greater attention toward holding perpetrators accountable. Indications of this trend include the increasing number of cases being prosecuted, the number of civil lawsuits filed against offenders, and the emergence of abuser registries.

But holding perpetrators accountable also requires that they be provided with opportunities to change their conduct, learn new behaviors, and make amends to victims and their communities. Professionals disagree about whether it is appropriate and desirable for APS, aging service providers, advocates, and others to work with perpetrators. Critics argue that with high caseloads, limited time, and insufficient resources, workers should focus on helping victims. Additionally, some believe that working with perpetrators can be damaging to their relationships with victims. There is also disagreement about the effectiveness of treatment for perpetrators.

Others point out that because many victims want to see their abusers helped, especially in the case of family members, it is neither antithetical nor damaging to work with abusers or see to it that they receive help. Further, with the extremely limited supply of caregivers, helping abusive caregivers to provide better care may be a cost effective use of workers' time. Some point out that because many inappropriate behaviors were learned, they can also be unlearned. Others, including proponents of restorative justice, family caregiver advocacy, and family reunification programs (see Chapter 3) believe that working with whole families, including abusive members, is the most effective way to stop abuse.

Because few services have been developed for abusers, service providers have looked to related fields, including mental health, domestic violence, and family caregiving for techniques and approaches. Although, for the most part, the following techniques are untested, they are believed to hold promise.

Counseling for Perpetrators

Counseling for perpetrators may focus on a variety of issues depending on the type of abuse, perpetrators' motives, and their willingness and ability to change:

- Breaking through Denial. Chapter 3 describes how perpetrators use "neutralization techniques" to rationalize, justify, and deny their actions and suggests that these techniques can be countered.
- Reality Testing. Abusers, like victims, may have unrealistic perceptions and expectations about the seriousness of abuse and their own culpability. Just as showing victims photographs of their injuries can break through denial, it may achieve the same effect with abusers. Reality testing with abusive caregivers may, for example, address caregivers' unrealistic expectations about elders' abilities and needs or counter their suspicions that care receivers are faking symptoms or are capable of doing more for themselves. This can be accomplished through education about aging and chronic illnesses.
- Exploring Past Relationships. When abusers have been victimized in the past by their victims or others, exploring their own

victimization may help them overcome anger and resentment, understand their actions, and develop empathy.

- Behavioral Therapy. This type of counseling focuses on changing negative or counterproductive behaviors such as anger, substance abuse, and violence. Perpetrators can learn to control their impulses by focusing on their own behavior, rather than that of their victims, and recognizing that although external stresses cannot always be controlled, the responses to these stresses can be. Other methods for achieving greater self-control include countering abusers' fatalism (e.g., the belief that they cannot control their actions), and abusers' tendency to blame others for their problems or unhappiness (Ganley, 1981).
- Establishing Clear Expectations. Practitioners can reach agreements or contracts with perpetrators to stop abuse or make amends. Provisions may include specific steps they will take to relieve stress and timelines for returning stolen items.
- Options Counseling. Abusers can benefit from educational materials and professional help to explore their options with respect to vocational training, support or treatment groups, and drug treatment programs (Ganley, 1981).
- Reducing Social Isolation. Helping abusers develop social skills, encouraging them to engage in social activities, and providing regular personal contact can increase abusers' self-esteem, decrease their frustration, and increase the chances that future abusive incidents will be discovered. Once abusers feel accepted and comfortable with practitioners, they may be willing to expand their circle of contacts to include others in the community.

Domestic Violence Treatment

A few elder abuse prevention programs have adapted techniques used in "batterers' treatment" programs for perpetrators of elder domestic violence. In addition, programs that serve abusers of all ages are increasingly serving perpetrators of elder abuse. Some of these programs are also starting special groups for elder abusers.

Participants are typically ordered into batterers' treatment by courts as a condition of probation, through diversion programs, or through negotiated plea agreements. The programs offer group and individual counseling that focuses on helping perpetrators learn to control violent impulses, improve their communication skills, assume responsibility for their actions, and gain insight into their attitudes about violence and women. Because batterers express a wide variety of negative feelings through anger, which leads to violence, some programs help perpetrators expand their "emotional repertoires" and find more appropriate ways to express frustration, worry, hurt, or embarrassment (Ganley, 1981; Sonkin & Durphy, 1982). Cognitive approaches used in battering treatment programs focus on helping perpetrators understand the role of men and women in society, and the use of power and control in intimate relationships.

Δ *The Stop Elder Abuse and Mistreatment Program (SEAM) of Lifespan, a nonprofit agency in Rochester, New York, offers a psycho-educational program for elder abusers modeled after domestic violence programs for batterers. The program assumes that many abusers are not psychopathological and can be educated to recognize their behavior as abusive and unacceptable. Participants may be court ordered into the sixteen-week program, or referred by APS, adult probation, and others in the legal or medical community. The program covers aging awareness, the myth of entitlement, issues of power and control, and taking responsibility for one's actions. A video of abuse scenarios is used as the basis for discussions. The program claims a 92% success rate; that is, 92% of perpetrators referred to SEAM stop their patterns of elder abuse. The program is not limited to spouses or by gender. (Doolity & Greenberg, 2003)*

The following comments are from Alan Silvia, the facilitator of a batterer treatment group that extended eligibility to permit elder abuse perpetrators to participate with other perpetrators of domestic violence:

> Most of the older men have never been in the criminal justice system before, and being labeled as a criminal or having an arrest record for the first time almost brings some of them to tears. They feel more pain at having their names in the paper, and depression plays a major role . . . Most are finally being arrested for things that they've been getting away with for 20, 30, 40 years.
>
> Some of the older men are in total shock when they're arrested. A case that really sticks out in my mind is one in which the police were called to the home of a man in his 70s. He was pushing and shoving his wife, and saying she was crazy. Here was a guy who could hardly walk and was partially blind, arrested for an act of domestic violence. It took a long time for him to accept the fact that he wasn't the victim. It's not uncommon for older batterers to believe that they are model citizens. Another thing that some older batterers can't understand is being removed from their homes on restraining orders. If the home belongs to them, they can't believe anyone has the right to take it away. It's totally unacceptable to them.
>
> The "blended groups" also work well because some of the attitudes are "catchy." Sometimes you see situations where a younger batterer

says, "Nobody's going to tell me what time I have to come home," and an older guy will say, "You don't know what you're talking about. How would you like having your wife come home at 10 o'clock at night? . . . When a batterer corrects another batterer or describes his life experiences, it has more of an impact than when it comes from a facilitator. You find younger people who appreciate the older men's experiences and understanding. So, I think there is some benefit in the wider range of ages. (Nerenberg, 1999)

Programs for Caregivers

Many practitioners assume that abuse by caregivers can be prevented or reduced by providing caregivers with services to reduce their stress and/or burden. Services for caregivers, which are described in Chapter 3, include information to help them understand diseases and their progression, instruction in managing difficult behaviors, respite, financial relief, and support groups.

Despite this assumption, few programs, services, or materials have been designed specifically for abusive or high-risk caregivers. An exception is a training program aimed at preventing caregiver abuse that was developed in the late 1980s at the University of Alabama (Scogin et al., 1989). Caregivers who were identified by mental health workers as being abusive or at risk for becoming abusive participated in training that was largely adapted from parenting programs and child and spouse abuse treatment programs. It covered the biopsychosocial aspects of aging, problem solving, stress and anger management, and utilization of community resources.

Educational materials and programs designed to help caregivers assess and reduce their risk of becoming abusive include the following:

Δ *The Office of Geriatric Medicine/Gerontology at Northeastern Ohio Universities College of Medicine developed Preventing Stress from Becoming Harmful: A Guide for Individuals Who Care for Persons with Dementia.*[10] *This guide helps caregivers assess their own level of stress, understand their own stress "triggers," and develop techniques for reducing stress and risk. It is available in English and Spanish.*

Δ *Preventing Elder Abuse by Family Caregivers Technical Assistance Manual.*[11] *Produced by the National Center on Elder Abuse, this guide provides consumers with resources, Web sites, recommended reading, and a list of things caregivers can do to reduce caregiver stress.*

Δ *A Fact Sheet on Caregiver Stress and Elder Abuse.*[12] *Also produced by the National Center on Elder Abuse, this fact sheet provides an overview of the problem of abuse by caregivers, red flags to look for, and things that can be done by agencies and community members.*

Little is known about the effectiveness of treatment programs for abusive caregivers and those at risk for abusing. Among the notable exceptions is an evaluation of an education and anger management program in the United Kingdom. The evaluation explored the program's effectiveness in reducing conflict among perpetrators of physical elder abuse and neglect. The study demonstrated a significant reduction in conflict among abusers but no significant changes among neglectors (Reay & Browne, 2002).

An evaluation of the training program for preventing caregiver abuse at the University of Alabama, which is described earlier in this section, explored the trainings' effectiveness in lowering risk (Scogin et al., 1989). Caregiver participants were compared with other caregivers with respect to factors that were believed to be associated with risk. These risks included "personal costs" associated with caregiving and symptoms of distress, anger, and low self-esteem. Participating caregivers experienced some reduction in the personal costs of providing care as well as a decrease in symptoms of distress, whereas nonparticipants experienced an increase. The training program had little impact, however, on anger and self-esteem.

CONCLUSION

Although it is clear that tremendous progress has been made in responding to the needs of elderly victims of abuse, their families, and abusers; it is equally clear that the development of services to prevent elder abuse is still a work in progress. Many communities lack the services and interventions described in this chapter. Strategies for expanding the pool of services and filling gaps are addressed in the next chapters. Chapter 6 describes what agencies, courts, and communities can do; and Chapter 7 describes state and tribal initiatives. As new programs are designed and launched, the need for research to measure their success and point the way to promising new approaches will become increasingly critical. Specific needs for program evaluation are addressed in Chapter 9.

NOTES

1. See http://www.ncea.aoa.gov/ncearoot/Main_Site/index.aspx.
2. For more on IDEAL, see http://www.bennettblummd.com.

3.For more on the Self-neglect Severity Scale, see the Web site of the Consortium for Research in Elder Self-neglect of Texas at http://www.bcm.edu/crest/.

4.For more information, see the IOA's Web site at http://www.ioaging.org/.

5.For more information on "It's MI Identity," visit the Web site of Michigan's attorney general at http://www.michigan.gov/ag.

6.NCCUSL is an organization of lawyers, judges, and law professors appointed by states to draft proposals for uniform and model laws and work toward their enactment.

7.Guardians are called conservators in some states.

8.For more information on the Center for Social Gerontology, see http://www.tcsg.org.

9.For more information, see http://www.tcsg.org/mediation/SJI_01.pdf.

10.For more information, see http://www.neoucom.edu/audience/about/departments/Gerontology/Resources.

11.Available online at http://www.ncea.aoa.gov/NCEAroot/Main_Site/pdf/family/caregiver.pdf.

12.Available online at http://www.ncea.aoa.gov/NCEAroot/Main_Site/pdf/family/caregiver.pdf.

CHAPTER SIX

What Agencies, the Justice System, and Communities Can Do

INTRODUCTION

One of the most fascinating aspects of my work has been seeing the remarkable ingenuity and creativity that professionals, agencies, and community groups have shown in tackling abuse and neglect. Often that involves taking good ideas from others and expanding, improving upon, or adapting them for diverse settings or populations. For many years, I have wanted to compile a list of the hundreds of practices and approaches that I have heard, read about, or tried. This chapter and the two that follow are a first effort at doing so. This chapter focuses on programs, services, policies, and innovations that agencies, courts, and community groups have developed; Chapter 7 focuses on state and tribal initiatives; and Chapter 8 is devoted to outreach, which may be carried out at the local, state, tribal, and national levels.

WHAT AGENCIES CAN DO

Even agencies with limited resources can improve their response to elder abuse. Through such simple measures as putting up an elder abuse prevention outreach poster or assigning an elder abuse "point person," agencies have conveyed to clients that they are concerned about the problem and prepared to respond. In doing so, they have encouraged victims and vulnerable seniors to talk about their situations or get the word out

Table 6.1   What Agencies Can Do to Stop Abuse

- Develop specialized elder abuse units or elder abuse "specialists"
- Participate on community-wide elder abuse multidisciplinary teams, councils, and task forces
- Provide information on elder abuse and reporting laws to all new employees as part of their orientation
- Provide in-service training to keep staff apprised of new developments in the field such as changes in their reporting responsibilities and new research findings
- Develop policies and procedures for handling abuse and neglect cases that:
  - Permit employees to work in teams when necessary
  - Allow adequate time for making comprehensive assessments, building rapport, and working at victims' pace
  - Establish clear agency guidelines for reporting abuse
  - Inform all elderly clients early on about the agency's reporting responsibilities
- Make information on abuse readily available through posters, pamphlets, or other educational materials in waiting rooms, restrooms, and offices
- Ensure that the staff who handle abuse cases have access to the support and tools they need; these may include
  - State-of-the-art interview protocols, assessment tools, and technology
  - Adequate support and supervision from managers
  - Access to legal advice
- Negotiate interagency agreements with other agencies involved in elder abuse prevention to improve coordination, collaboration, and communication
- Develop prevention services

---

to others. Other agencies have made abuse prevention a top priority and devoted significant resources to prevention.

The ideas and practices described in this section are divided into two sections: general practices that can be implemented by any agency and those that are appropriate for specific types of agencies, settings, or disciplines.

General

The following practices can be implemented by any agency or institution that serves elders (see Table 6.1 for a summary):

- Develop specialized elder abuse units or elder abuse "specialists." Elder abuse cases require highly specialized knowledge and skills. Because the field is evolving rapidly, staying abreast of new developments can also be a formidable challenge. Large agencies, including police departments and prosecutors' offices, have responded by creating specialized elder abuse units, whose members focus primarily or exclusively on abuse cases and receive special training to help them build their skills and expertise. Small agencies with limited resources have designated "elder abuse specialists" to either handle all the elder abuse cases that the agency receives or to consult with, assist, and train others to work with victims. Elder abuse specialists may also assume responsibility for representing their agencies on interagency teams, planning councils, or other forums to inform the public and other professionals about their agencies' abuse prevention services. Elder abuse specialists or members of specialized units are usually provided with opportunities to attend conferences or other training events and, ideally, assigned smaller caseloads in light of their added responsibilities and the labor-intensive nature of many abuse and neglect cases.

- Participate on community-wide elder abuse multidisciplinary teams, councils, and task forces. Agencies can support representatives' participation and maximize the benefits by asking them to give reports at staff meetings, at managers' meetings, or through in-house memos or newsletters.
- Provide information on elder abuse and reporting laws to all new employees as part of their orientation. Information should be included in orientation manuals or packets and covered in orientation sessions. New employees can be asked to sign statements verifying that they have received and read the information.
- Provide in-service trainings to keep staff apprised of new developments in the field such as changes in their reporting responsibilities and new research findings.
- Develop policies and procedures for handling abuse and neglect cases that:
  - Permit employees to work in teams when necessary. This may include making joint home visits with colleagues within or outside the agency. The benefits and reasons for working in teams vary. Some cases can benefit from the expertise of more than one discipline, whereas, in others, it may be helpful to have one partner focus on victims' needs and the other, on abusers' needs.
  - Allow adequate time for making comprehensive assessments, building rapport, and working at victims' pace. This may require smaller caseloads or the relaxing of rules that limit the number of visits workers can make or the length of time they can keep cases open.
  - Establish clear agency guidelines for reporting abuse and designate someone to make decisions when conflicts or differences of opinion arise with respect to reporting.
  - Inform all elderly clients early on about the agency's reporting responsibilities. Doing so can reduce the risk of future conflicts

if workers need to report. It also provides an opportunity to raise the issue in a nonthreatening way, which may encourage some victims to disclose abuse. It further conveys the message that the agency is concerned about abuse, knowledgeable, and prepared to help.

- Make information on abuse readily available. Agencies can place abuse prevention posters, pamphlets, or other educational materials in waiting rooms, restrooms, and offices.
- Ensure that the staff who handle abuse cases have access to the support and tools they need. These may include
  - State-of-the-art interview protocols, assessment tools, and technology
  - Adequate support and supervision from managers
  - Access to legal advice
- Negotiate interagency agreements with other agencies involved in elder abuse prevention to improve coordination, collaboration, and communication. Agreements should provide for joint investigations, assessments, and care planning when appropriate. Agreements should also address issues of confidentiality and information sharing.
- Develop prevention services. Specific areas of need include daily money management, information about frauds and scams, advice about advance directives, and support services.

Agency-Specific Practices

The following steps can help specific agencies or disciplines improve their response.

APS Programs

Cases referred to APS programs have become increasing complex, requiring highly specialized expertise in clinical, legal, and financial matters. To meet the challenge, APS programs have instituted a variety of measures. These include

- Upgrading the staff prerequisites or competency standards for new employees
- Instituting more rigorous processes for investigation, risk assessment, and case substantiation to ensure that elder abuse victims are adequately protected
- Assigning individuals or subunits to specialize in certain types of abuse cases.

Δ *APS workers in San Francisco are assigned to one of five units. Members of the "financial abuse unit" work closely with police officers in the city's fraud unit and receive special training in handling complex cases. Workers in the "high risk unit" monitor and assist "repeat clients" and those who are ambivalent about receiving help or otherwise in need of special attention.*

- Providing specialized consultation and technical assistance for employees. APS programs are providing personnel with specialized consultation in such areas as cognitive assessment, forensics accounting, undue influence, and geriatric medicine. Some programs contract with individual consultants on an ongoing or as-needed basis. Others have collaborated with universities, hospitals, or other agencies to provide expertise. And some have recruited volunteers with special expertise.

  Δ *Oregon's Department of Human Services hired a full-time forensics nurse to assist in investigations. The department also established the Retiree Response Technical Team (R2T2), which recruits and trains retirees with expertise in financial affairs to help APS workers investigate financial abuse cases and participate on multidisciplinary teams.*

  Δ *Under a pilot project conducted by Temple University's Institute on Protective Services, forensic accountants are available to APS agencies and others in Pennsylvania to assist with financial abuse investigations, write reports, and serve as expert witnesses.*

  Δ *In Texas, subject experts are available to help with APS investigations of financial abuse and self-neglect.*

Other measures that APS programs have initiated include:

- **Staff development.** Highly advanced training programs have been developed for new and experienced workers. The National Adult Protective Services Association (NAPSA) maintains a database of training materials, which include Web-based training programs, curricula, videos, and Power Point presentations on a broad array of topics including self-neglect, ethical issues in APS, forensic accounting, investigation in long-term care facilities, guardianship, and many more.[1]

- **Technological innovations.** APS programs are providing workers with new tools for maintaining records, collecting evidence, staying in touch with supervisors and experts, keeping track of offenders, and sharing information.

  Δ *The Texas Department of Family and Protective Services provides APS workers with tablet personal computers and digital cameras to use in the field. Workers are also provided with an automated, multidomain, risk assessment tool.*

- **Registries:** Some states have established registries of abusers, including family members, paid caregivers, and others. The registries can be accessed by potential employers, criminal justice professionals, or others.

  Δ *Missouri maintains an employee "disqualification list" of persons who have misappropriated funds or property of residents in long-term care facilities.*

Domestic Violence Programs

Domestic violence programs have improved their response to elderly victims by assigning elder abuse specialists and collaborating with aging and elder abuse prevention programs to conduct outreach campaigns. Some have trained staff in how to work with elderly victims and modified shelters to make them more "elder friendly."

Δ *The Women's Center of Bloomsburg, Pennsylvania, designated one of its domestic violence counselors as the "Elder Abuse Counselor" to work with the local APS program and enhance coordination between the domestic violence and aging services communities. The counselor, who went through an intensive APS training program, accompanies APS staff on home visits when domestic violence is believed to be occurring. She talks to the victims while APS representatives work with the alleged abusers. The Women's Center has also developed safe homes for elder victims who need emergency shelter (National Center on Elder Abuse, 1996).*

Health Care Facilities

Personnel in doctors' offices, hospitals, clinics, home health care agencies, and other health and medical facilities are often the first, and may be the only, professionals with whom victims have contact. As such, they play a crucial role in seeing to it that victims receive help. Specific steps some have taken include the following:

- Screening all elderly clients for elder abuse and neglect. The American Medical Association has promoted this practice by developed a short list of screening questions (American Medical Association, 1992).
- Encouraging or requiring personnel to use forensic medical protocols, forms, or procedures.

- Developing in-house protocols for handling abuse cases.
  - Several hospitals have developed protocols to assess potential abuse and determine when cases need to be reported to authorities. Examples include the Mount Sinai/Victim Services Agency Elder Abuse Project in New York, Beth Israel Hospital in Boston, and Harborview Medical Center in Seattle.

Providers of Home Health Care

Because home health care clients are likely to spend long periods of unsupervised time with their workers, the need for stringent screening, training, and monitoring of workers is crucial. Providers of home health care have instituted the following measures (Nerenberg, 2002).

- **Enhanced screening for employees.** Usually, agencies and programs determine potential employees' suitability for employment and eliminate unskilled ones by using written applications, personal interviews, and references supplied by applicants. A few agencies check applicants' state criminal records. Supplemental steps that can enhance safety and eliminate unscrupulous candidates include checking federal criminal databases, child and dependent adult abuse registries, motor vehicle records, sex offender registries, and, in the case of licensed professionals, disciplinary board records.
- **Consumer education.** Seniors and family members who hire their own workers should be instructed in how to find, screen, and monitor them. Some organizations have published "tips" to reduce the risk of abuse, which include securing elders' valuables, requiring receipts for purchases made by helpers, employing more than one worker (with alternating shifts), closely monitoring bank accounts and phone bills, and keeping important financial information and documents locked up. Some organizations encourage family members to make unannounced visits.
- **Codes of conduct or ethics.** The sustained and often intimate contact engendered by the caregiving relationship can lead to a blurring of the boundaries between personal and professional conduct. Clients who develop close relationships with their helpers may want to give them gifts, help them with personal problems, loan them money, or become romantically or sexually involved. Persons who rely on others for their basic necessities are further susceptible to undue influence, exploitation, and subtle forms of coercion. Codes of conduct or ethics can clarify

appropriate conduct with respect to privacy, confidentiality, gifts, and personal or sexual relations. Codes also need to provide guidance to employees in what to do if their clients or clients' family members engage in inappropriate, illegal, unsafe, or disturbing conduct.

Legal Service Providers

Legal aid programs for the elderly have traditionally offered consumer protection, public benefits counseling, tenants' rights advocacy, assistance with advance planning for health care and finances, and other legal matters. Now, programs are increasingly developing expertise in such areas as predatory lending, restitution advocacy, annulling bogus marriages and adoptions, restraining orders, home repair scams, and other forms of abuse. Special initiatives include the following:

- Recruiting private attorneys and law students to serve on referral panels or assist clinics on a pro bono or reduced fee basis (Kristof, 2006)
- Conducting outreach and educational programs that focus on crime prevention and the legal rights of older persons
- Ensuring that the social service needs of clients are met by offering legal and social services in tandem. This can be done by pairing attorneys with social service providers within agencies or through interagency collaboration.
  Δ *Legal/Social Service Elder Abuse Prevention (LEAP), a program operated by the Jewish Association for Services for the Aged in New York City, pairs lawyers with social workers to provide elderly victims of domestic violence with social and legal services, including safety planning and orders of protection.*

Dementia Care Programs

Dementia care programs can reduce the risk of elder abuse and increase the likelihood that those who abuse or are abused as a result of dementias are provided with appropriate prevention and treatment services. Specifically, these programs can do the following:

- Provide training to their staff in elder abuse, including the relationship between elder abuse and caregiver stress, reporting, and resources offered by protective service programs (for more on the training needs of various professional groups, see Chapter 9)

- Adapt existing clinical assessment protocols to "red flag" high-risk factors and situations (Nerenberg, 2002c):
  - Caregivers who may be at heightened risk include those who
    - Have been violent in the past
    - Fear they will become violent
    - Suffer from low self-esteem
    - Perceive that they are not receiving adequate help or support from others
    - Have compromised mental and physical health
    - Perceive caregiving responsibilities as a burden
    - Are experiencing emotional and mental "burnout," anxiety, or severe depression
    - Feel "caught in the middle" by providing care to children and elderly family members at the same time
  - Care receivers who may be at heightened risk include patients who
    - Are verbally or physically aggressive, combative, or abusive
    - Engage in disturbing behaviors
    - Need high levels of help with ADLs and IADLs
  - The risk of abuse is also heightened when caregivers and care receivers
    - Live together
    - Had a poor relationship prior to the onset of the illness or disabling condition
    - Are married or intimate partners, and have a history of conflict or domestic violence

Dementia care programs can take the following additional steps to reduce risk and ensure an appropriate response when abuse is discovered:

- Work with law enforcement personnel to help them recognize elders who are violent or disruptive as a result of dementias and provide training in how to work with them.
- Develop new (or adapt existing) counseling programs for groups or individuals that address the emotional or mental health needs of abusive or high-risk caregivers. These counseling programs could address the following issues:
  - Depression and low self-esteem
  - Current and past conflicts between family members
  - Caregivers' expectations of care receivers
  - Caregivers' expectations of themselves
  - Negative attitudes about caregiving
  - Alcohol and substance abuse

- Fear of becoming abusive
- Develop education materials and programs that focus on the following needs, issues, and problems:
  - Community services, how to access them, and resources to pay for them
  - Techniques for responding effectively to care receivers' disruptive and aggressive behaviors, including violence, combativeness, and embarrassing conduct in public
  - How to determine the need for long-term care services
  - How to select, hire, and monitor long-term care providers and facilities
  - Empowering care receivers to participate in decision-making about their care.

Some measures that have been developed by dementia care programs include the following:

Δ *The Wisconsin Alzheimer's Association sends teams across the state and country to conduct training to law enforcement in how to work with people with dementias.*

Δ *The Buffalo (New York) Alzheimer's Association chapter teaches recruits at the police academy how to recognize dementia patients and defuse conflicts.*

WHAT THE JUSTICE SYSTEM CAN DO

Communities have improved the justice system's response to elder abuse by shoring up existing services and resources, and by starting new programs. They have enhanced the response of law enforcement agencies, prosecutors' offices, victim witness assistance programs, and courts; they have also developed new agencies and court-based programs. Following are some examples of the approaches and innovations they have implemented.

Law Enforcement

As police and sheriffs' departments encounter more elder abuse cases, many have developed units that specialize in working with elders or elder abuse cases. In addition to responding to reports of elder abuse and neglect, members of specialized police units may do the following:

- Provide liaison with APS and other community agencies
- Provide training to health and social service agencies in how to report criminal abuse
- Conduct crime prevention sessions for seniors' groups
- Routinely review abuse cases that are reported to APS, long-term care (LTC) ombudsmen, or others to identify criminal conduct
    Δ *In Milwaukee, Wisconsin, the police department has created a Senior Citizen Unit called the "Gray Squad," which includes five detectives, eight uniformed officers, and a uniformed sergeant. Everyone assigned to the squad receives sensitivity training on working with elderly victims and are familiarized with community resources. The Gray Squad responds to personal crimes against seniors, including assault, robbery, personal larceny, confidence crimes, and other frauds. The unit collects data from incident reports to identify patterns that can help focus prevention and intervention initiatives.*

Prosecutors' Offices

Prosecutors' offices have improved their response to abuse through the following measures:

- Creating specialized units that include attorneys and victim/witness coordinators with special training.
- Implementing policies and approaches that reduce trauma and hardships for elderly victims, including "fast-tracking" and "vertical prosecution." Fast tracking avoids lengthy delays in court-related hearings, and vertical prosecution is where one attorney handles the same case and victim from beginning to end. This minimizes the number of times the elderly victim has to recount the details of the assault (Heisler & Stiegel, 2002).
- Creating cross-agency response teams to accommodate special needs. For example, elder sexual assault teams may include advocates and nurse examiners, who both meet with victims at the same time.
- Developing forensic examination rooms and offices equipped with closed-circuit telecommunication with courts and creating comfortable, easily accessible interview rooms on secure floors.
    Δ *San Diego County's Elder Abuse Prosecution Unit includes prosecutors, criminal investigators, and an elder advocate. The advocate uses elder-sensitive response protocols and procedures for evidence collection that were designed to*

reduce trauma to elderly victims. The advocate checks all police reports daily and follows up with victims over sixty-five, and the unit works with hospital emergency rooms to improve detection of elder physical abuse. Members of the unit also speak at banking conferences to heighten awareness about financial abuse, monitor "boiler rooms," and make frequent visits to retirement communities to make presentations on crime prevention. They also transport victims to and from court appearances.

Victim Advocacy Programs

Victim advocacy programs have designated special advocates to work with elders, carried out outreach campaigns, provided training to staff in the special needs of elderly victims, and developed policies and procedures to improve access. Victim advocates can enhance victims' experiences in the criminal justice system and improve case outcomes through the following:

- Respond to elderly victims' need for special assistance to attend meetings and court-related hearings
- Alert police and prosecuting attorneys about elderly victims' special needs so that they can be considered in scheduling police lineups, filing charges, holding hearings, and so on
- Provide information and assistance to victims, their families, and service providers, including
  - Helping victims complete applications for compensation and obtaining medical information, bills, police reports, and so on
  - Providing security measures and protection against witness intimidation and harassment
  - Providing referrals for services for victims, including mental health care, support groups, temporary or permanent housing, home repair, and safety checks of victims' homes
- Work with victims' informal support networks and social service providers to help them understand the traumatic impact of crime, including victims' tendency to become isolated and blame themselves
- Keep victims apprised when offenders are arrested or released and help them take extra security precautions as needed
- Protect victims from publicity by escorting them to and from courtrooms, and, in particularly sensitive cases, asking judges to close courtrooms to the public

- Promote measures to ensure that victims of financial crimes enjoy the same rights as victims of violent crimes
- Develop large print referral cards that provide information on victims' rights and services

Forensics Centers

Forensic centers bring together experts and use state-of-the-art science and analytic tools to study and respond to illegal conduct that is usually associated with social problems. They provide diagnostic resources to identify wrongdoing, support law enforcement, and conduct research and training.

 Δ *The first forensic center designed exclusively for elder abuse was launched in 2003 as a partnership between ten organizations in Orange County, California, including the University of California, Irvine's College of Medicine, APS, the DA's office, and local police and sheriffs' offices. It is staffed by professionals from legal, medical, social service, and law enforcement agencies who investigate evidence, review cases, conduct in-home medical and mental status assessment, and interview victims. The Center also provides education, consultation to other professionals, and research in such areas as bruising and pressure ulcers.[2] In 2006, Los Angeles County started a similar center.*

 Δ *San Francisco's Consortium for Elder Abuse Prevention has developed a "virtual forensics center." A network of experts is available to provide free online and telephone consultation to local agencies in such areas as capacity and undue influence. The program also offers free geriatric assessments.*

Elder Justice Centers

Family Justice Centers house police, prosecutors, forensic experts, and victim advocates from public and private nonprofit agencies in the same building to provide "one-stop shopping" and "wraparound" services for victims.

 Δ *San Diego's Family Justice Center, which has been widely replicated in the United States and Canada, joined forces with the San Diego District Attorney's Office in 2006 to extend services to victims of elder abuse. A Family Justice Center in Waterloo, Ontario also developed specialized services for abused elders.*

Casey Gwinn, founder of the San Diego Family Justice Center, had this to say about the Center:

The benefits of having all the services in one place go beyond the convenience factor. DAs, victim advocates, police, APS . . . we all think in silos. But you can't get away that when you work together in the same office every day. You have to deal with the differences and learn to work together. It also generates a synergy.

The approach is also empowering to victims. We had an elderly client, Wanda, who was the victim of fraud. She was incredibly ashamed of what had happened to her. When she met with an advocate from the DA's office, a volunteer advocate, a detective, and an APS worker, she couldn't believe that all these people wanted to help her. She even came to team meetings where we discussed her case. The district attorney successfully prosecuted her abuser, who has agreed to pay restitution after his release from custody. Wanda wanted to pay us. She couldn't believe our services were free.

Improving Court Access

Coming to court poses special problems for frail elders. Whether coming to testify, seek protective orders, or for other matters, they often experience long waits, have to stand in line, or find it difficult to navigate physically. In addition, compromised mobility, memory, vision, and hearing may make it even more difficult to participate in court proceedings (Rothman, Dunlop, & Seff, 2006).

Courts have attempted to overcome these obstacles by becoming more "senior friendly." They have made physical modifications and procedural changes to improve access, which include designing safe and comfortable waiting areas, instituting special calendars, and assigning court staff to provide extra assistance to elders.

> Δ *Stetson University College of Law's Centers for Excellence in Elder Law and Advocacy are working together to create the first elder-friendly courtroom. Everything in the courtroom has been designed to be user-friendly for the elderly and disabled.*[3]
> Δ *San Diego has a special "senior waiting room" at the courthouse that has oxygen and wheelchair accommodations.*

Elder Courts

A few communities have developed special "elder courts" to meet elders' special needs:

Δ *Hillsborough and Palm Beach Counties (Florida) have developed "elder courts," which employ case managers to explain the court system to victims, describe what will happen to perpetrators, arrange for transportation or court accompaniment, request victim compensation, and, when necessary, assist in making special arrangements such as videotaping testimony. The case managers also maintain an extensive directory of community services and make referrals, following up to ensure that clients' needs are met. In addition, victims are given help to complete court documents such as protective orders, and court personnel monitor guardianships. Legal forms are also reproduced in large typeface.*

Δ *Alameda County's (California) Elder Protection Court was established in 2002 featuring a separate calendar (in the late morning) for elders seeking restraining orders. In some situations, when elders are unable to appear in court, the proceedings are conducted in chambers, with a judge issuing orders by telephone. Court clerks offer extra help to those filling out petitions for elder abuse protective orders, and those seeking orders do not have to wait the usual twenty-four hours to obtain a judge's signature. Instead, clerks personally deliver requests to the judge, who reviews them immediately. To obtain longer-lasting protective orders, seniors must return to court several weeks later for hearings. In the meantime, a case manager interview elders, other family members, and, in many cases, abusive relatives or caregivers. The case manager also makes referrals to community agencies, runs criminal background checks, arranges transportation to court hearings, and sets up telephone hearings for housebound or hospitalized elders. In January 2006, the court's role was expanded to include a criminal docket.*

Self-Help Clinics

Self-help clinics and services provide access to courts by people who cannot afford lawyers or who lack access for other reasons. Examples include self-help clinics for obtaining orders of protection and for helping family members and friends who want to become guardians.

Δ *In 2005, San Francisco's Probate Court started a no-fee, self-help clinic to provide information to prospective conservators of person, inform them about alternatives, and help them fill out forms.*

Guardianship Monitoring

For many years, significant attention has been paid to the lack of court oversight of guardians to ensure that they do not abuse those they have been entrusted to help. Whereas some courts actively investigate proposed guardians, routinely monitor those that have been appointed, and intervene when guardians abuse, neglect, or do not act in the best interest of those they are appointed to serve, others exercise minimal control. A 2004 survey of three states conducted by the Government Accountability Office found that only one-third of the courts tracked guardianship appointments (GAO, 2004). The remaining courts did not know how many appointments had been made, were often unable to determine if required reports had been submitted, and frequently could not document the status of wards.

The findings of a national 2005 study of court practices in guardianship monitoring by AARP and the American Bar Association (Karp & Wood, 2006) were equally troubling. Of the 387 respondents—who included guardians, probate judges, court managers, elder law attorneys, and legal representatives of people with disabilities—over 40% reported that no one was assigned by courts in their jurisdictions to visit individuals under guardianship and only one-fourth said that someone visits regularly. The report further identified ways that monitoring could be improved, which include heightened accountability with respect to required reports and accounts by guardians, visits to individuals under guardianship, the use of technology in bolstering monitoring, guardian training, court-community collaboration, and increased funding.

Communities have developed a variety of programs to monitor guardianships, which range from court-operated programs staffed by highly trained professionals to informal programs that use volunteers. Although the programs vary in terms of their methods, resources, and effectiveness, they typically recruit individuals with backgrounds in social work, accounting, finance, bookkeeping, and the like. These individuals report to the court concerning the well-being of wards and the status of their assets. They also ensure that court-required reports are accurate and submitted on time.

The GAO report cited above identified several exemplary court-based guardianship monitoring programs. In addition to requiring guardians to receive training and file reports, the programs that were highlighted used volunteers to visit wards:

Δ *In Tarrant County, Texas, social work students visit wards to fulfill their internship requirements. A licensed Master Social Worker on the court staff acts as program manager and trains and supervises the interns. The students receive course credit, and there are typically four or five interns making an average of sixty to seventy visits each month. The visitors submit a report of their visits to the program manager for review, and the judges subsequently review the reports to guide their decisions on whether to continue the guardianships.*

Δ *In Rockingham County, New Hampshire, the court recruits volunteers, primarily retired senior citizens, to serve as researchers or to visit incapacitated people, their guardians, and care providers at least annually, and to submit reports of their findings to court officials. The researchers prepare files for the court with contact information, case background, and the last annual guardian's report. The visitors then contact the guardians and arrange to visit the incapacitated person. They assess the wards' living situations, finances, health, and social activities, and recommend follow-up actions to the court. A court employee serves as the volunteer coordinator.*

Other entities, besides courts, may operate guardianship monitoring programs. Examples include the following:

Δ *Guardianship Services Inc. (GSI), a private nonprofit agency in Texas, recruits, trains, and supervises volunteers who serve as guardians for residents of skilled nursing facilities. Volunteers visit patients on a weekly basis; make medical, placement, and end-of-life decisions; and manage the finances of those they supervise.*

Δ *In Idaho, Volunteer Guardian Boards recruit and select volunteers and meet monthly to consider wards' cases.*

WHAT COMMUNITIES CAN DO

Recognizing that elder abuse is a community problem that calls for a community response, groups around the country have developed multidisciplinary teams, coalitions, planning councils, task forces, and other partnerships to improve coordination and spearhead outreach, advocacy, and resource development. Specific activities are described in the following sections.

Multidisciplinary Teams

Multidisciplinary teams (MDTs) have become a hallmark of elder abuse prevention, highlighting the fact that no single agency has all the resources, services, or expertise needed to handle all forms of abuse in all settings. Teams provide a forum for professionals from diverse disciplines and agencies to discuss difficult abuse cases; learn what services, approaches, and resources are available from other agencies and disciplines; share information and expertise; identify and respond to systemic problems; and ensure offender accountability. MDTs typically include health and social service providers, law enforcement personnel, LTC ombudsmen, mental health care providers, physicians, advocates for persons with developmental disabilities, lawyers, domestic violence advocates, money managers, case managers, and many others.

In the last decade, specialized teams have emerged to address specific forms of abuse (Teaster & Nerenberg, 2003; Nerenberg, 2004).

Financial Abuse Specialist Teams (FASTs)

The first Financial Abuse Specialist Team (FAST) was organized in Los Angeles when local service providers acknowledged the need for specialized expertise to help abuse investigators distinguish fraudulent from legitimate financial transactions, prevent losses, build cases for court, and recover misappropriated assets (Aziz, 2000). Since then, many other communities have started FASTs. FASTs recruit members with expertise in real estate, insurance, banking practices, investments, trusts, estate planning, financial planning, and other financial matters. Because some forms of financial abuse fall under federal jurisdiction, the teams are also likely to include representatives from state and federal law enforcement and regulatory agencies, including attorneys general, U.S. attorneys, and the Federal Bureau of Investigation. FASTs have also been actively involved in providing training to other professionals in their communities and advocating for new services and policy.

Rapid Response FASTs

Professionals in Santa Clara County, California, developed a variation of the FAST model to respond to financial emergencies, which include situations in which abusers have access to elders' funds, when thefts or fraudulent transactions are about to be committed, or when a quick response is needed to preserve evidence (Malks, Buckmaster, & Cunningham, 2003). Unlike traditional FASTs, which can be quite large, Santa Clara operates five small teams, each of which includes an APS social worker, a public guardian investigator, a district attorney investigator, and a deputy county attorney. The teams respond to financial emergencies within a few hours, or by the next day in nonemergencies. All cases are reviewed by APS workers who conduct joint investigations with other FAST members. APS workers may conduct joint investigations with public guardian investigators when elders have diminished mental capacity, or with district attorney investigators when it is likely that crimes have been committed. The county attorneys get involved when civil actions are needed such as securing restraining orders to prevent sales and filing actions for breach of fiduciary duty, fraud, negligence, and unfair business practices.[4]

Fatality (Death) Review Teams

Patterned after child and domestic violence fatality review teams, elder fatality review teams explore unexplained deaths of elders, distinguish "natural" deaths from homicides and murders, shed light on events leading up to deaths, identify systemic problems, instruct members in how to evaluate injuries and causes of death, and aid in prosecution. Teams typically include coroners, medical examiners, health care and social service providers, law enforcement agencies (local, state, and, in some situations, federal), prosecutors, and representatives from state agencies that oversee long-term care facilities. Some fatality review teams include morticians, funeral home operators, and hospice care workers. Mental health professionals may also provide guidance in evaluating the predeath mental state of decedents to look for signs of suicide as well as interpreting clients' cognitive status at an earlier period in time.

In 2002, the Commission on Law and Aging of the American Bar Association received funding from the U.S. Department of Justice Office for Victims of Crime to promote the development of local and state-level elder death review teams. The ABA developed a replication manual and provided technical assistance to teams around the country (Stiegel, 2005). The California Medical Training Center has also developed a replication manual for teams within California.

Geriatrician Diana Koin, who serves on death review teams in Sacramento and San Mateo Counties and authored the California Medical Training Center's replication manual, offers the following fictional case example, patterned after an actual case, and comments.

> An emergency response technician, responding to a 911 call, found a 92-year-old woman lying on the floor of her home, which she shared with her daughter. She had been there for hours, incontinent, and unable to get up. Emergency room personnel tested her blood, which showed that she was dehydrated and malnourished. She also had pressure ulcers and died a few days later from sepsis of the ulcers. The ER reported the case to APS, which referred it to the death review team. The daughter claimed that her mother had refused care.

In cases like these, we usually start by reviewing elders' histories. Often, as in my example, patients' capacity at the time of death and leading up to death is critical because others are claiming they refused help. So we look for indicators of incapacity in their histories. We also often discuss "systems" issues such as who should have made reports and when, or whether the LTC ombudsman's mandate against reporting to the police without victims' consent also prevents them from asking police to perform "well-being checks." The prosecutor on the team tells us what information and evidence she needs to build cases.

Sometimes, we've had cases that everyone originally thought were abuse, but turn out not to be. For example, we reviewed a case that involved a man who died from complications of multiple fractures associated with neglect and possible assault. We were puzzled because the patient's history failed to show any past history of abuse. On closer examination, it turned out that the recorded cause of death was incorrect and that he had actually died from metastatic cancer that had spread widely to his bones.

Medically Focused Teams

A few multidisciplinary teams have been organized to provide medical expertise to APS and other community agencies in abuse cases. Examples include the following:

Δ *The Vulnerable Abuse Specialist Team of Orange County, California (VAST) includes geriatricians, nurses, pharmacists, psychologists, medical social workers, psychiatrists, medical students, family practice residents, and others (Mosqueda, Burnight, Liao, & Kemp, 2004). Because most cases are referred by APS, the team conducts its weekly meetings at APS' offices and invites APS workers to participate. Other referrals come from police and prosecutors, and many of the requests that the team receives involve cases in which legal action has been taken. Team members evaluate injuries, signs of neglect, and cognitive functioning; interpret medical evidence or testimony; and provide court testimony. Members also provide training and education to medical residents and other health care providers, and conduct home assessments.[5]*

Δ *The Texas Elder Abuse and Mistreatment (TEAM) is operated by the Baylor College of Medicine, the Harris County Hospital District, and the Texas APS program. Clients referred to TEAM may be evaluated in an outpatient clinic setting, the hospital, or in their homes. TEAM has shared its expertise with communities throughout the state, and has been involved in clinical, education, and research projects. Because self-neglect cases are among the most commonly referred cases, TEAM members have joined with other faculty from Baylor and other academic institutions to form the Consortium for Research in Elder Self-neglect of Texas (CREST) to further explore the condition.*[6]

Coalitions and Councils

Coalitions, planning and oversight councils, and task forces have emerged in communities around the world to improve their response to abuse. Some were formed by groups of professionals, whereas others were created through grassroots advocacy, appointed by public officials, or created by statute. These groups, which may include professionals, members of the public, or both, have tackled a wide range of problems.

Identifying and Responding to Unmet Service and Training Needs

Groups have identified the need for new services or training through formal needs assessments, public forums, or informal focus groups or discussions. They may respond to unmet needs through the following:

- Meeting with governmental or private funding sources to alert them to service gaps or unmet needs
- Crafting new service programs or appealing to existing programs to extend coverage to unserved or underserved groups
- Endorsing funding proposals developed by community agencies that want to start needed programs or provide training. This may require establishing review processes and criteria to ensure that proposed projects meet community needs, are cost-effective, and are likely to succeed.

Advocating for New Policy

Community groups and coalitions have met with local, state, and national legislators and their staff to alert them to the need for new services and policy. Some have conducted hearings or summits and helped to draft and enact new laws.

Improving Interagency Coordination

Community coalitions, councils, and task forces have improved coordination and cooperation between agencies by doing the following:

- Organizing and convening multidisciplinary teams
- Developing interagency protocols that establish the roles, responsibilities, and relationships among various agencies
- Advocating for public policy that facilitates coordination such as state laws permitting multidisciplinary teams to share information and reporting laws that provide adequate coverage and protection.

*Sponsoring Community Awareness and
Education Campaigns and Events*

Community groups have raised awareness about elder abuse, instructed elders and their families in how to avoid abuse, and provided communities with information about abuse prevention techniques and services. Several national organizations have sponsored or supported educational forums to their local chapters. AARP, for example, has developed comprehensive educational materials for local AARP chapters or individual members on consumer fraud. For a comprehensive discussion of community outreach campaigns, see Chapter 8.

Δ *The Big Sky Prevention of Elder Abuse Program in Billings, Montana, has, for several years, hosted an annual "Rubber Duck Regatta," a fund-raising event for families that includes music, children's' games and contests, and the duck races. The proceeds are used for the Senior Executive Financial Assistant (SAFE) program, which provides representative payee services and elder abuse training to professionals.*[7]

Volunteer Programs

Many communities are using volunteers, including retired professionals, students, elders who have been victimized themselves, and concerned citizens to accomplish the following:

- Provide specialized consultation to elder abuse workers and organizations. Retired professionals, including judges, police officers, financial specialists, and nurses, have provided specialized expertise to APS programs, other community agencies, and multidisciplinary teams. An example is the Retiree Response Technical Team (R2T2), which was described earlier in this chapter.
- Provide direct services to abused and vulnerable elders. Elders, including past victims, and other concerned citizens are serving as daily money managers, guardians, guardian monitors, peer counselors, friendly visitors, and support group facilitators.

- Advocate for systems' reform. Volunteers are supporting needed policy by contacting politicians, testifying at hearings, and hosting events. Some are monitoring courts to observe how they are handling abuse cases. Student interns are helping with needs assessments and other research.

  Δ *Ohio's Court Watch Project educates older adults about the court system and organizes groups to attend trials involving elder abuse. An investigator with the attorney general's office works with volunteers from AARP chapters, Retired Senior Volunteer Programs, and TRIADs.*

  Δ *Sonoma County's (California) Elder Abuse Prevention Council created a Court Advocacy Workgroup made up of senior volunteers. The group follows cases of elder abuse and exploitation to help raise the visibility of these cases within the judicial system.*

  Δ *The Florida Department of Elder Affairs' Senior Companion Program trains volunteers in abuse, neglect, and exploitation and in how to work with self-neglecting elders.*

  Δ *In Billings and Cascade Counties, Montana, Ameri-Corps*VISTA volunteers organized elder abuse prevention coalitions.*

  Δ *Volunteers are increasingly being used to monitor guardians. Examples are provided in the Guardianship Monitoring section of this chapter.*

WHAT COMMUNITY INSTITUTIONS CAN DO

Financial Institutions

Employees of financial institutions are often the first to observe financial abuse. For that reason, elder abuse prevention professionals have enlisted their aid in preventing elder financial abuse. In addition, financial institutions and trade associations have launched their own initiatives. Specific measures they can take include the following:

- Develop policies and protocols for handling suspected abuse. For example, banks may instruct tellers and supervisors to take the following steps when abuse is suspected.
  - Steps for tellers
    - Attempt to learn the reason for large transactions or frequent withdrawals. Ask elders (not those accompanying them) the reason for the change in activity.

- If persons accompanying elders or acting in their absence claim to have authority; check documentation, including signature cards, powers of attorney, and the like, as it is common for perpetrators to make false claims about their authority.
- Contact supervisors immediately if abuse is suspected. Together, the teller and supervisor can review account histories, patterns, and the transactions in question to determine if they should be processed, stopped, or reported to bank security or senior bank officers.
- Steps for supervisors
  - Speak to elders alone if they suspect abuse.
  - Warn customers about the dangers involved in carrying, withdrawing, or wiring large amounts of cash or of potential fraud.
  - Notify senior officers of questionable transactions.
  - Notify law enforcement if the elder is believed to be in immediate physical danger.
  - Consider delaying the transaction and confer with legal counsel or senior bank officers if customers are in immediate danger.
- Provide training to employees on the indicators and risk factors associated with financial abuse, how to report abuse, techniques for interviewing older customers, and community resources.
- Conduct regularly scheduled visits and offer limited banking ser vices at places convenient to older people, including senior centers and congregate living facilities.
- Take a proactive approach to developing new procedures and product lines, including the following:
  - Mechanisms for detecting unusual account activity
  - Alerts on accounts
  - Procedures for verifying suspicious transactions
  - Protected accounts for seniors
- Conduct customer outreach programs to alert elders to abuse and the protective measures they can take. Activities may include developing and distributing educational materials alerting elderly customers to scams and how to recognize the potential for elder financial abuse, conducting senior seminars or other presentations on elder financial abuse, and generating media attention on the issue of elder financial abuse and its prevention.
- Develop alliances with victim service providers, law enforcement agencies, and elder rights advocates.
- Permit staff to participate in elder abuse prevention activities or in groups such as multidisciplinary teams or financial abuse specialist teams (see FASTs).

- Develop "advance directives" giving financial institutions permission to report suspicious bank activity to local authorities, including APS or law enforcement. After explaining financial exploitation to new customers, elders are asked if they would like to sign directives. These directives remain in place even if elderly customers lose their ability to give consent. The directives address financial institutions' concern that reporting breaches customers' trust and confidentiality.

  Δ *The Massachusetts Executive Office of Elder Affairs developed the first "bank reporting project" in collaboration with the state's Executive Office of Consumer Affairs, the attorney general's Elderly Protection Project, and the Massachusetts Bank Association. Together, the partners developed procedures and guidelines for reporting and investigating abuse. The project also provided training for the staff of financial institutions and informational materials for customers.*

  Δ *The Elder Financial Abuse Prevention Program is a public/ private partnership, which includes the Oregon Bankers Association, the Oregon Department of Justice, AARP Oregon, the Oregon Association of Area Agencies on Aging, and the Oregon Department of Human Services. Together, the organizations produced a "kit" for bankers, which includes a manual and video to help bank personnel recognize and report possible elder financial exploitation. The video contains scenarios based on actual events that occurred in Oregon banks. The kit also includes a manual and video that provide instruction to banks in how to conduct seminars for seniors. It has been sent to every bank branch in Oregon.*[8]

  Δ *The Elder Financial Protection Network has developed a video on elder financial abuse that has been distributed nationally. It shows bank tellers how to spot potential abuse and what steps to take to prevent abuse from occurring.*[9]

  Δ *In Dane and Sheboygan Counties, Wisconsin, the sheriffs' departments, health and human service departments, and the district attorneys' offices collaborated on a community-wide project in which account holders at multiple banks can sign "advance orders to disclose." The orders give financial institutions authority to contact responsible parties (designated by the account holder), family members, or local law enforcement if any "unusual" banking transactions, such as large or frequent withdrawals, occur with the customers' accounts. The forms are available at local banks, savings and loans, credit unions, the offices of estate planners, attorneys, accountants, financial planners, nursing homes, and*

senior-living centers. They can also be obtained at the county's
health and human services and sheriff's departments, local police
stations, and on the county's Web site.

Δ *The California Bankers Association has developed a free, com-*
puter-based training program to help employees recognize the
signs of financial elder abuse, protect customers, and meet their
mandatory reporting requirements.[10]

Academic Institutions

Institutions of higher education are playing an important role in preventing abuse. Some are conducting practice-focused research and evaluations. Others are collaborating with APS and other community agencies
to develop training curricula, provide training, and consult in cases.
Still others have evaluated public policy related to abuse prevention and
assisted in developing new or improved policy. In addition, training in
elder abuse has been provided to students in schools of gerontology, social
work, criminal justice, business, communications, nursing, medicine, and
many more. Colleges and universities are also providing interns and volunteers to support program initiatives at the state and local levels.

Δ *The Texas Elder Abuse and Mistreatment Institute (TEAM) at*
Baylor College of Medicine (BCM), the first state adult protec-
tive services–medical school collaboration in the United States, is
involved in clinical, education, and research projects.

Δ *The Protective Services Training Institute is a partnership*
between the Texas Department of Protective and Regulatory Ser-
vices (PRSI) and four graduate schools of social work in Texas.
It provides state-of-the-art, interactive, skills-based training to
department employees who work in the states' adult and child
protective service, child care licensing, and intake programs.
The institute also has a certification program for workers and
researches and develops new training technologies.[11]

Δ *Several law schools around the country are offering securities arbi-*
tration and mediation clinics for low- and moderate-income victims
of investment fraud whose losses are too small to interest securities
lawyers. The cases are prepared by second and third year law stu-
dents under the supervision of seasoned lawyers. In some cases, the
students represent the investors at hearings (Kristof, 2006).

Δ *The Government Law Center at the Albany Law School researched*
statutes pertaining to durable powers of attorney around the
country and developed a list of recommendations for reform that
were used to develop laws in New York and other states.

Δ *The Jacob Reingold Institute for the Prevention of Financial Elder Abuse at the Brookdale Center on Aging of Hunter College conducted a study in 1994 that identified a need for financial management services to prevent or stop financial abuse. The study also revealed impediments to agencies providing the service. In response, the Institute began providing information and technical assistance to agencies on how to start and administer programs.*

Δ *Fordham University collaborated with the New York City Department for the Aging and the Mayor's Office to Combat Domestic Violence to develop and test a multidisciplinary training curriculum on domestic violence against older women in several jurisdictions including New York City. The project was funded by the United States Department of Justice (DOJ).*

Churches

Religious leaders can play an integral role in the lives of elder abuse victims and can have a very strong impact on preventing, detecting, and resolving elder abuse (Podnieks & Wilson, 2003). A 2000 study at the University of Toronto surveyed faith leaders, two-thirds of whom indicated that they were aware of abuse taking place within their congregations.

Δ *The Communities Against Senior Exploitation (CASE) Partnership, developed by the Denver District Attorney's Office is a partnership between the DA's office and faith-based organizations to provide community-based services for elder financial fraud prevention, intervention, reporting, and victim support. In its first two years of operation, CASE partnered with 225 churches, synagogues, and other entities. Project personnel presented fraud prevention workshops and send fraud alerts to partnering congregations, which inserted them in bulletins.*

CONCLUSIONS

Agencies, interagency coalitions, and community groups around the world have mobilized communities to accommodate elderly victims' special needs, coordinate their efforts, build consensus about how to best serve abused elders, and promote public policy that supports and facilitates service delivery. Despite this progress, much remains to be done. Creating effective community responses to elder abuse is not limited to launching new programs and services, but rather, must include sustained and systematic efforts to monitor the system, evaluate new programs and policy, and respond to new needs. The challenges they face in doing so are explored further in Chapter 9.

NOTES

1.For more information, see http://www.reft.org/TA/NAPSA/catalog/catalog.htm.

2.For more information, see the center's Web site at http://www.centeronelderabuse.org.

3.See http://www.law.stetson.edu/Eleazercourtroom/.

4.A free video describing the Santa Clara FAST is available from the Office for Victims of Crime. Information is available on OVC's Web site at http://www.ojp.usdoj.gov/ovc/publications/infores/other.htm.

5.For more information on VAST and the Center of Excellence, see http://www.centeronelderabuse.org.

6.For more information on CREST, see http://www.bcm.edu/crest/.

7.For more information, see http://www.mtelderabuseprevention.org/projects.html#SAFE.

8.For more information on the Oregon materials, see http://www.oregonbankers.com/community/efapp/.

9.For more information, see http://www.bewiseonline.org/index.shtml.

10.For more information, see http://www.calbankers.com/content/fea.asp.

11.For more information on Texas's Protective Services Training Institute, see http://www.utexas.edu/research/cswr/psti/.

CHAPTER SEVEN

What States and Tribes Are Doing

INTRODUCTION

With little guidance from the federal government, states and tribes in the United States have taken the lead in developing systemic responses to elder abuse. They have mandated or encouraged professionals and the public to report suspected cases of abuse, set up response systems, funded APS and other services, assessed needs, improved the response of the civil and criminal systems, and taken steps to ensure that professionals have the training and tools they need to respond effectively. Some states have gone further in developing comprehensive strategic plans.

This chapter provides examples of public policy and activities that were spearheaded by state and tribal governments, agencies, and coalitions. The list is not exhaustive, but rather, provides a sampling of trends and promising practices. It begins with what states are doing, followed by tribal initiatives. Public awareness campaigns are covered separately in Chapter 8.

WHAT STATES ARE DOING

States' initiatives to improve their response to elder abuse are organized according to the goals they were created to accomplish.

Ensuring that Professionals Report and Respond Appropriately

Preventing elder abuse requires that professionals and the public recognize abuse and know what to do when they encounter or suspect it. It further requires that once cases are identified they are investigated by trained professionals and that the parties involved are offered services to stop abuse, prevent its recurrence, or treat its effects. To achieve these objectives, reporting laws need to be clear, and the response needs to be timely, uniform, and well coordinated.

As described in Chapter 3, reporting laws are the foundation of state elder abuse prevention programs. In most states (44), the duty to report is mandatory, which means that people in certain jobs, settings, or professions must report. Those typically covered include health and mental health care providers, caregivers, social service providers, nursing home employees, and virtually anyone who works with elders. Voluntary reporting laws encourage professionals and the public to report. All states provide immunity from liability for those reporting in good faith (Moskowitz, 2003).

Most states have designated APS as the agency to investigate reports in both private homes and long-term care facilities and to provide support and referrals to victims. Other agencies play primary or supportive roles depending on the type of abuse, the setting in which it occurs, and whether it constitutes criminal conduct. In some states, for example, LTC ombudsmen have responsibility for investigating abuse in long-term care facilities. Other agencies that may have roles to play when abuse occurs in long-term facilities are Medicaid fraud control units, which are authorized to prosecute patient abuse and mistreatment in facilities that receive Medicaid funds, and agencies that license and oversee long-term care facilities.

Abuse reporting statutes vary widely, but typically they do the following:

- Define elder abuse and neglect and establish what types of abuse are reportable
- Define the circumstances in which victims are eligible for services and what services are provided
- Provide protections for reporting parties and penalties for failure to report and knowingly making false reports
- Define what agencies have responsibility for investigating reports and providing services
- Establish the roles, relationships, and responsibilities of local and state agencies, including provisions for the cross-reporting of cases

- Provide for data collection that permits intra- and interstate evaluation
- Provide due process protections for alleged abusers

Although little is known about the impact of reporting laws, the number of reports received by APS has risen by 30% in the past ten years (Teaster, Lawrence, & Cecil, 2007), which suggests that reporting has been successful in bringing cases to light. States are also increasingly extending coverage to include new professional groups. Recent additions in some states include bank employees, clergy, animal care and control workers, and coroners.

But as states gain experience with reporting laws and response systems, they have encountered new problems, needs, and challenges. Many mandated reporters fail to report, and problems with coordination among APS and the other agencies involved in investigating and responding are frequently reported (Rosenblatt, Cho, & Durance, 1996). As cases become more complex and the potential consequences for alleged abusers become more severe, APS and other agencies involved in the reporting process need guidance in how to substantiate claims, protect the rights and privacy of both victims and abusers, prevent abusers from reoffending, and manage programs effectively.

Lack of compliance with reporting laws has been attributed to many factors. Among these are mandated reporters' failure to recognize abuse, a lack of awareness about the reporting process, a fear of becoming involved in legal proceedings or having to appear in court, a fear of arousing the anger of abusers, and concerns about confidentiality (Moskowitz, 2003).

State lawmakers have attempted to improve compliance by adding penalties for failure to report, clarifying definitions, and addressing the training needs of reporters. Some require that all mandated reporters receive training, whereas others require training for certain groups or for certain types of abuse. For example

Δ *Iowa requires that all mandated reporters receive two hours of training relating to the identification and reporting of dependent adult abuse within six months of initial employment (or self-employment) and at least two hours of additional training every five years (Iowa Code § 235B.16). The state also has a panel to review and approve mandated reporter training curricula.*

Revisions to states' reporting laws are also increasingly addressing the management of APS programs. They are, for example, adding or modifying policies and procedures in many areas including quality control, program oversight, disclosure of client information, time frames for investigations, case substantiation, and confidentiality. Some states have also created registries of offenders and due process protections for offenders.

Problems in coordination often stem from a lack of clarity with respect to the roles, responsibilities, and relationships among those involved in the reporting process, as well as concerns about information sharing and confidentiality. To improve coordination, states have revised or added provisions about cross-reporting, notification, and referral among APS, LTC ombudsmen, law enforcement, medical examiners, and others. Some states have also authorized or encouraged APS programs to develop or participate on multidisciplinary teams and allowed for the sharing of information among team members. Because state statutes covering elder abuse may appear in multiple sections of state codes—including guardianship laws, penal codes, and health and safety codes—states are increasingly cross-referencing reporting laws with other statutes and addressing variations in definitions.

Ensuring Justice

As more abuse cases reach the criminal and civil justice systems, states are addressing the myriad problems involved in holding offenders accountable and ensuring victims' rights.

Improving Prosecution Rates

Experts and professional associations have identified a variety of problems and challenges involved in building criminal cases (American Prosecutors Research Institute, 2003; Heisler & Stiegel, 2002; Morgan & Scott, 2003). They include the following:

- A lack of training for police, prosecutors, and judges
- Victims who are unwilling or unable to participate in the criminal justice process
- A shortage of forensics experts and information
- A lack of sufficient resources and personnel for law enforcement agencies and prosecutors' offices to marshal evidence, locate witnesses, and secure expert witnesses
- A lack of clarity with respect to roles and responsibilities because elder abuse cases may fall under local, state, or federal jurisdiction or because, in some instances, jurisdiction may be overlapping

States have responded to these problems and others and attempted to enhance prosecution rates by creating special offenses, enhancing sentences, relaxing evidentiary rules, and using other methods.

- Creating Special Offenses. As described in Chapter 5, many forms of elder abuse correspond to "traditional" crimes like assault, battery, domestic violence, attempted murder, theft, larceny, or extortion. Some states, however, have created special offenses that reflect the special relationships victims are likely to have with their abusers, their heightened vulnerability, the greater impact crimes are likely to have on them, and the obstacles they are likely to face in seeking justice. For example

  Δ *California Penal Code § 368 contains provisions concerning physical, mental, and financial elder abuse. Three of its major provisions are (1) anyone who knowingly allows or inflicts unjustifiable physical pain or mental suffering on an elder is guilty of a felony or misdemeanor; (2) care providers who willfully cause or permit elders to be placed in situations where their health is endangered are guilty of felonies or misdemeanors; and (3) predators may face sentence enhancements if victims suffer great bodily harm or death.*

- Enhancing Penalties. Other states have also enhanced penalties in certain situations (National Center for Victims of Crime, 1999):

  Δ *In Nevada, offenders who commit crimes against persons over the age of sixty are subject to a prison term twice as long as that normally allowed for the same offense.*

  Δ *Louisiana law mandates that all violent crimes against the elderly be punished by a minimum of five years imprisonment with no opportunity for parole.*

  Δ *Georgia imposes an enhanced penalty for unfair or deceptive business practices directed toward the elderly.*

- "Relaxing" Evidentiary Rules. The U.S. Constitution guarantees criminal defendants the right to be confronted with the witnesses against them. For that reason, out-of-court statements, called *hearsay*, are generally not permitted because those making them are not available for cross-examination. Some states have modified their rules in light of special obstacles that elder abuse cases pose (see below).

In the past, when victims of domestic violence failed to appear in court, judges commonly dismissed the cases. As domestic violence was better understood, courts stopped dismissing criminal charges solely on the basis of a victim failing to appear. Instead, they permitted the use of compelling out-of-court testimony. This includes recordings of calls to 911 and "spontaneous declarations" (or "spontaneous utterances"), which are statements made by people when they are upset or under stress, and which are considered to be reliable.

Victims of elder abuse are also likely to recant their stories or refuse to testify. Some are unable to come to court because of declining health or disability. To overcome these obstacles, some states have permitted the use of videotaped or out-of-court statements by elders (Meyers, 2005; Moskowitz, 2003).

In 2004, however, the Supreme Court issued a warning to states about relaxing evidentiary rules regarding hearsay through the *Crawford v. Washington* decision. The case involved the assault conviction of Michael Crawford, who was convicted of stabbing a man he believed had tried to rape his wife. The court barred the tape-recorded, eyewitness account of the stabbing by Crawford's wife, ruling that "testimonial statements" made out of court cannot be used at trial unless the person who made the statement is available for cross-examination. Statements are considered "testimonial" if they are knowingly made to law enforcement or government agents associated with law enforcement and provide evidence for later use at court (Meyers, 2005).

This decision has severely restricted the use of evidence that was previously admissible. However, the long-range effects of the ruling are not known. The court did not define the various types of testimonial statements that are covered, and new cases are testing the decision. Lower courts, for example, have been trying to resolve when 911 calls can be used when callers are not available to testify (*Davis v. Washington*).

- Other states have enacted a variety of other provisions, including expedited trials and the extension of statutes of limitations, to increase the prosecution rates of elder abuse offenders.
  - Δ *Delaware allows for the extension of the statute of limitations for a period of up to three years beyond the normal five-year limitation for felonies when "an offense is committed as one in a continuing course of conduct of offenses involving forgery, fraud, falsification or tampering with records, breach of fiduciary duty, theft, or misapplication of property," and the offense was discovered after the passing of the normal limitation time (Delaware Code § 205, Title 11).*

Encouraging Civil Attorneys to Handle Abuse Cases

Civil attorneys have historically been reluctant to handle elder abuse cases. Many victims are unable to pay private attorneys; judges may not award attorneys fees; and, because compensatory damages are based on life expectancy and earning power, they are significantly lower for elders than for younger clients (Moskowitz, 2003). In addition, pain and suffering claims do not survive the death of the plaintiff in most tort cases. This raises concerns that the plaintiffs will die or become incapacitated before the cases are settled (in which case, lawyers may not get paid). The slow pace of the legal system further increases that risk. Cases are also difficult to prove as a result of victims' being unwilling or unable to come to court or testify, delays in discovering that abuse has occurred, and a shortage of expert witnesses.

These problems have prompted some states to pass laws that make it more practical for elderly victims to file civil suits and for lawyers to represent them. California was the first state to pass a law that makes it more financially viable for lawyers to represent elderly victims in civil lawsuits (Hankin, 1996). Passed in 1992, the Elder Abuse and Dependent Adult Civil Protection Act allows for postmortem recovery for pain and suffering and mandates attorney fees and costs (Cal. Welf. & Inst. Code §§ 15600-15657.3).

Other states have also made elder abuse cases more economically feasible through the following measures:

- **Increasing damages.** These provisions vary widely in terms of the situations in which they apply:
  Δ *Georgia law doubles civil damage awards if it is shown that the perpetrator specifically targeted elderly victims (Ga. Code Ann. § 10-5 B-6[c]).*
  Δ *Illinois law authorizes treble damages for losses incurred by an elderly or disabled person as a result of financial exploitation when the exploiter is criminally charged and fails or refuses to return the victim's property (720 ILCS 5/16-1.3).*
  Δ *In Arizona, persons in positions of trust and confidence who violate their duties are subject to civil damages up to three times the amount of the monetary damages and forfeit their claims on the elders' estates (Ariz. Rev. Stat. § 46-455).*
  Δ *In Nevada, if an older person suffers personal injury or death caused by abuse or neglect or suffers a loss of money or property by exploitation, the offender may be ordered to pay up to two times the actual damages incurred. If the offender acted with recklessness, oppression, fraud, or malice, the court must order the person to pay the attorney's fees and costs of the person who initiated the lawsuit (NRS 41.1395 1).*
- **Modifying standards of proof.** The standard of proof typically applied to elder abuse cases in the civil justice system is "clear and convincing" evidence. Some states have changed the standard used in some cases to "preponderance of evidence," which is easier to meet.

- **Expedited handling of cases.** Some states have expedited the handling of civil cases under certain circumstances. For example
  Δ *Colorado provides for earlier trial dates when a party suffers from an illness or condition that raises a medical doubt of survival beyond one year or if the person is age seventy or older and can prove to the court that he or she has a meritorious claim and a substantial interest in the case (Ridgway, n.d.).*

Extending Victim Compensation and Assistance to Elders

As described in Chapter 3, many elderly victims of crime or abuse do not receive victim compensation or assistance. The Office for Victims of Crime, which administers Victim of Crime Act (VOCA) compensation and assistance funds, acknowledged the need to improve access to these funds for elderly crime victims (U.S. Department of Justice, Office for Victims of Crime, 2002b). In response, the federal guidelines that dictate how states can use VOCA funds were revised to permit and encourage states to extend eligibility for compensation to elders who report to APS only (they were previously only available to victims who cooperated with law enforcement). Under the revised guidelines, victims who have experienced financial, as well as violent, crimes are eligible for services, including mental health assistance and support groups, credit counseling and advocacy, and restitution advocacy.

The extent to which states have taken advantage of these changes is not known. According to the National Center for Victims of Crime, as of 2005, only six states had modified their state laws or procedures to allow VOCA compensation funds to be used for services to financial crime victims (Deem, Nerenberg, & Titus, 2007).

States have, however, taken other steps to benefit elderly victims, which include the following:

- Waive minimum loss and deductible provisions for compensation for elders. Many victim compensation programs have "minimum loss standards" ranging from $100 to $200, which preclude claims for lesser amounts, or they require victims to absorb the first $100 or $200 of their losses. Recognizing that even small losses can be a hardship for people on fixed incomes, some states have waived these provisions for elders (National Center for Victims of Crime, 1999).
- Although many programs will not compensate victims for the loss of personal property, some states have created an exception when the property lost is considered essential to elderly crime victims (such as eyeglasses, dentures, hearing aids, or other medical equip-

ment). A few states have even compensated home-bound victims for the loss of their television sets or radios (National Center for Victims of Crime, 1999).
* Create outreach programs to the elderly to educate them about compensation.
  Δ *Illinois has enlisted the aid of librarians to help older victims of crime and abuse apply for resources under the Illinois Crime Victim's Compensation Act. Seminars are offered for community outreach librarians to increase their awareness of the needs of older victims, to increase their understanding of victims' legal rights and options, and to facilitate community connections with local elder rights advocates.*

Addressing Problems with Restitution

Restitution is when criminal courts order perpetrators to repay victims for money or property losses incurred as a result of crimes. Although many victims have a legal right to restitution, and restitution is among the most highly valued rights of many crime victims, few elderly victims receive it for a variety of reasons (U.S. Department of Justice, Office for Victims of Crime, 1999). Judges often fail to order restitution and, when they do, may underestimate the amount of losses. Also, because most criminal cases are settled without trials, sentencing judges frequently have limited information about the crimes, including the amount of money or property lost by victims. Additionally, victims who are not officially included in formal indictments are ineligible to receive restitution unless their repayment is part of a plea negotiation.

Perhaps the most commonly cited barrier to restitution is the fact that many perpetrators have spent the money, placed assets in the names of others, or hidden assets. As a result, victims usually collect a fraction of what they are owed. Other problems associated with recovery include the fact that most restitution payments begin after defendants are released from custody, which may be years later. It may further be unclear who is responsible for ascertaining victims' losses and enforcing restitution.

The federal government has acknowledged these and other problems associated with restitution and encouraged states to improve collection and distribution. In January 2005, the U.S. General Accounting Office (GAO) released *Criminal Debt: Court Ordered Restitution Amounts Far Exceed Likely Collections for the Crime Victims in Selected Financial Fraud Cases.* The report revealed that of the cases it reviewed, only 7% of the ordered restitution had been paid despite the fact that the defendants had reported significant wealth or assets prior to their judgments. The report recommends that asset forfeiture measures be taken earlier in investigations and prior to sentencing, and encourages prosecutors to place more pressure on offenders to pay off all restitution and fines prior to sentencing as part of plea agreements. It further calls for aggressive collection and fair distribution of restitution (GAO, 2005).

States are addressing the problems of restitution through policy reform and special programs. Examples include:

Δ *In California, restitution for medical and psychological treatment is mandatory for victims of assault, assault with a deadly weapon, or battery who are over the age of sixty-five.*

Δ *Rhode Island mandates restitution for breaking and entering the dwelling of an elderly victim.*

Δ *The Juvenile Court in Louisiana may distribute unclaimed restitution to elderly victims of nonviolent crimes for whom restitution has been ordered but not paid.*

Δ *In Vermont, victims are paid restitution from a government fund that is generated by a 15% state surcharge on criminal and traffic court fines. The Vermont Center for Crime Victims Services administers the program, assumes the debt, and collects from offenders. In this way, trained professionals, rather than individual victims, are the ones tracking down perpetrators' assets. Furthermore, victims do not need to wait months or years to collect; they are paid up to $10,000 from the fund immediately after their abuser is sentenced. The approach is also fairer because historically, victims who could afford to hire lawyers were the most likely to collect restitution.[1]*

Δ *In 2003, Oregon passed SB 617, which requires courts to order full restitution when the state presents evidence to support a victim's loss, injury, or damages. In addition, it states that the restitution is due and payable at the time of the judgment. This is a change from the previous law, which allowed the courts to consider the defendants' ability to pay before ordering restitution. It acknowledged that restitution should be ordered based on the loss to the victim, not on a defendant's ability to pay at the time of sentencing.*

Δ *Colorado conducted a pilot project in which courts employed collections investigators to ensure that victims received court-ordered restitution. A review of the state's restitution statutes also led to revisions, which include the requirement that criminal restitution be considered after conviction for any felony, misdemeanor, petty offense, or traffic misdemeanor offense (USDOJ, 2002).*

Δ *In Dakota County, Minnesota, the probation department allows probationers to pay off restitution by doing community service. Offenders work for minimum wage, and the county pays victims from a restitution fund (Murray & O'Ran, 2002).*

Ensuring a Comprehensive, Coordinated Service Response

Exploring Needs

States have explored unmet needs for services and policy by conducting legislative hearings, convening summits, and commissioning studies. Coalitions or politicians have spearheaded some of these initiatives, whereas others were in response to criticism leveled against agencies that are charged with responding to abuse reports.

Δ *Michigan's Task Force on Elder Abuse, which was established by Governor Granholm in 2005, developed one of the country's most comprehensive (Walker, 2005). Led by the Michigan Office of Services to the Aging, the task force studied statewide initiatives concerning elder abuse across the country and developed sixty recommendations covering a wide range of issues.[2] The report includes detailed rationales for each recommendation and estimates the costs associated with its implementation. Among the recommendations are the following:*

Δ *Create a statute to provide that durable powers of attorney (DPAs) be registered, prior to use, on a Web-based registry. The statute would also require agents to sign an acknowledgment of duties informing them of their responsibilities. The DPA would then be validated with a Certificate of Registration.*

Δ *Require financial institutions to read a disclosure to customers who want to create joint bank accounts and have them sign an acknowledgment disclosing the true nature of the account*

Δ *Adopt the Uniform Securities Act in a form that treats annuities as securities and regulates them under the authority of the State Securities Commissioner*

Δ *Establish an educational and advocacy campaign about annuities fraud*

Δ *Establish public/private partnerships with unions and other groups representing nonlicensed direct care workers to enhance awareness of elder abuse, develop appropriate courses of action when union workers identify cases of elder abuse,* and investigate the willingness of union officials to report elder abuse when workers are unable or unwilling to come forth individually

Δ Require that transactions benefiting caretakers (including conveyances and estate plans) above a certain amount be prepared and witnessed by disinterested attorneys (to reduce the risk of undue influence)

Δ Authorize expedited, ex parte financial protection orders

Δ Ensure that home appraisals are accurate, that appraisers do not inflate property values, and that lenders do not influence the appraisal process

Δ Establish an automated system that selects appraisers from panels

Δ Amend Michigan's appraiser licensing code to sanction appraisers who inflate or manipulate appraisal values

Δ Establish an in-home care regulatory and education study committee comprising public and private stakeholders to review existing laws/regulations, make recommendations, and provide oversight of the implementation of those recommendations. The committee will also identify and review outcome measures to prevent or reduce the risk of elder abuse, neglect, and exploitation by individuals and business organizations providing in-home services of any kind, particularly those agencies that are not certified by Medicare or Medicaid.

Δ In August 2000, the Wisconsin Department of Health and Family Services launched the Adult Protective Services Modernization Project. The project was designed to examine the state's APS services, elder abuse reporting system, and other laws and regulations, and to recommend ways to improve the state's response.[3]

Δ In 2004, Texas Governor Rick Perry ordered an investigation of the state's APS program. The investigation following a series of negative media stories about elders living in deplorable conditions. These elders had been repeatedly referred to the agency, but had apparently been lost in the system. The investigation revealed the need for increased funding to hire adequate employees and improve training (Mixson, 2005).

Δ Following the National Summit on Elder Abuse (convened by the National Center on Elder Abuse in 2001 to develop a national plan of action for elder abuse), Oregon and New York sponsored statewide summits. Following the Oregon event, Governor Ted Kulongoski assigned a task force to develop a statewide plan. The group developed comprehensive recommendations and urged the governor to implement the following measures:

Δ *Expedite criminal background checks for employees of long-term care facilities and other people who work with vulnerable populations; provide closer supervision to new hires until the checks are finalized; and create a list of disqualifying crimes to be used in "fitness determinations" for applicants*

Δ *Explore the development of a registry of individuals who have committed abuse against vulnerable adults*

Δ *Assign the Department of Corrections to develop a system to notify managers of long-term care facilities when predatory sex offenders are placed in facilities and establish a standardized referral process*

Δ *Urge the Department of Human Services to work with the Oregon Medical Association and the Oregon Nurses Association to develop a list of qualified experts to serve as expert witnesses in elder abuse criminal cases*

Δ *Urge the Oregon Health and Science University (OHSU) to convene a broad-based panel of experts to discuss the identification and classification of pressure ulcers to help in the successful prosecution of criminal abuse or neglect cases*

Δ *Encourage academic institutions and community groups to develop standardized information to educate guardians and conservators and to discuss the development of statewide standards for guardians and conservators*

Δ *Encourage the state-wide expansion of community-based volunteer programs (like AARP's Money Management Program) to help protect lower income vulnerable adults*

Improving Interagency Collaboration and Coordination

States have fostered collaboration and coordination among agencies and departments that provide elder abuse prevention services by creating incentives for working together, facilitating multidisciplinary teams, and developing protocols and memoranda of understanding that define working relationships.

Δ *When Wisconsin's Bureau of Aging and Long Term Care Resources received an increase in elder abuse direct service funds, counties were told that to receive the additional funds, they had to (1) have or develop an interdisciplinary team, which should include representation from a local domestic violence program; and (2) provide evidence of ongoing collaboration with domestic violence programs (Raymond, 2002).*

Δ *The Oregon Attorney General's Task Force on Elder Abuse coordinates policy and related issues regarding elder abuse and neglect.*

Δ *California passed legislation authorizing the establishment of elder death review teams. The law eliminated confidentiality barriers by allowing for the exchange of information among members (California Penal Code §§ 11174.4–11174.9).*

Protecting Elders with Diminished Capacity and Those at Risk for Undue Influence

States have taken a variety of approaches to protect elders with diminished capacity and those susceptible to undue influence. They have provided detailed definitions of capacity; addressed the critical shortage of guardians and other surrogates, particularly for elders with limited assets; and instituted guardianship reform measures.

Clarifying Capacity and Undue Influence

As described in earlier chapters, mental capacity and undue influence are critical considerations in elder abuse cases. Among the complexities that service providers face are defining capacity for specific tasks and proving when elders have been unduly influenced. Examples of measures that states have taken to help include the following:

Δ *California's Due Process in Competency Determination Act, enacted in 1996, provides guidance to courts in determining what mental functions are needed to make specific legal decisions, including contracting, conveying, marrying, making medical decisions, executing wills or trusts, and other actions. The law is based on a "presumption" of capacity, which means that it assumes that people have legal decision making capacity until or unless it is proven that they do not. It further assumes that having a deficit alone does not affect this presumption and that judicial determinations of incapacity cannot be based on diagnoses alone (e.g., a diagnosis of Alzheimer's disease). The statute lists "mental function deficits," including alertness and attention, the ability to process information, etc., which are also listed on the state's Capacity Declaration for Conservatorship.4 The statute further specifies that incapacity determinations must demonstrate how deficits correlate with the acts or decisions in question (Cal Probate Code §§ 810-814).*

Δ *Maine's "Improvident Transfers of Title" statute involves the transfer of real estate for "less than full consideration." Typically,*

*plaintiffs have had the burden of presenting evidence to support
their claims that defendants exercised undue influence. The new
statute created a presumption that the transfer was the result of
undue influence in certain situations and placed the burden to
prove they did not use undue influence on defendants (Me. Rev.
Stat. Ann. Tit. 33 § 1022).*

Increasing the Supply of Guardians

Although the impact of widespread shortages of guardians has not been
formally assessed, anecdotal evidence suggests that impaired individuals
who lack guardians or other surrogates are at risk of becoming homeless, impoverished, dependent, or debilitated. Some are institutionalized
unnecessarily.

Guardians include family members and friends; private, nonprofit
agencies; public guardians; and private professionals. The shortage of
guardians for people with limited assets stems from problems involving the first three groups (Quinn & Nerenberg, 2005). Barriers that discourage family members and friends from serving as guardians include
difficulties securing bonding, lack of information, and the associated
expenses, which may include attorneys' fees.

The shortage of private, nonprofit agencies willing to provide all
forms of money management, including guardianship of estate, has, in
part, been attributed to concerns about liability. Some agencies have
encountered difficulties finding affordable insurance that provides
adequate protection against staff errors, omissions, or malfeasance.
Concerns about liability are heightened by obstacles that agencies face
in screening employees. Laws that were created to protect workers' privacy make it difficult for employers to obtain information on employees' past work experience, histories of abuse, or criminal backgrounds.
Providing guardianship is also costly and labor intensive. For example,
in some situations, guardians must be available twenty-four hours a
day to respond to emergencies. And, because agencies for the elderly
are strongly committed to preserving clients' freedom and autonomy,
some are understandably reluctant to provide a service that is typically
involuntary.

The public guardianship system is particularly overburdened
(Teaster et al., 2005). Public guardianship has been defined as "the
appointment and responsibility of a public official or publicly funded
organization to serve as legal guardian in the absence of willing and
responsible family members or friends to serve as, or in the absence of
resources to employ, a private guardian" (Teaster et al., 2005). Factors
that contribute to the shortage include the heightened demand that has

resulted from the increase in the old-old population. Another factor is that public guardians have experienced reductions in revenue. This has been attributed by some, in part, to the growing number of private professional guardians who typically serve incapacitated clients with assets. In the past, public guardians were more likely to serve some wards with assets (guardians are entitled to request reimbursement for their services).

Examples of approaches that states have employed to address the shortage of all forms of guardians include the following (Quinn & Nerenberg, 2005):

Δ *Virginia has encouraged family members and friends to serve by passing legislation that provides for petitioners to be reimbursed for costs and fees from the estate. The reimbursement is paid even if the guardian is not appointed as long as the court finds that the petition was brought "in good faith and for the benefit of the respondent."*

Δ *Contra Costa (California) County has a conservatorship workshop where family members who want to serve or who are currently serving as conservators can get help.*

Δ *Texas enacted legislation that permits agencies that serve as guardians to charge a portion of their fees to Medicaid clients. The fees are deducted from the clients' share of cost for nursing home care.[5]*

Δ *Florida uses unclaimed funds from the estates of wards to extend the resources of its public guardianship program. The funds are held by the state treasurer for five years and then deposited in the Department of Elderly Affair's trust fund to be used for the benefit of public guardianship.*

Δ *Illinois has a two-tiered public guardian system in which the county public guardians serve individuals with estates over $25,000 and the state guardian serves those with estates of $25,000 or less.*

Δ *In Massachusetts, incapacitated nursing home residents needing guardians sued the state Medicaid agency. The court ruled that a medical guardian was an essential prerequisite for providing medical care to a resident unable to give informed consent to treatment, and therefore, Medicaid must allow a medical or remedial deduction for such care (Rudow v. Commissioner of the Division of Medical Assistance [Mass., No. SJC-07760, March 11, 1999]).*

Ensuring Accountability by Guardians

Problems associated with guardianship and public guardianship have been widely acknowledged by the media, Congress, the Government Accountability Office, and national organizations. These groups and other forums have identified widespread abuses of the personal liberties of wards, a lack of standards for guardians, and the absence of court monitoring (Quinn, 2005). The rapid growth of the field of private professional guardianship, which is largely uncontrolled and unregulated, has been the cause of particular concern.

States have implemented a variety of measures to assure greater accountability by guardians. Resources that have been developed to help them include the National Probate Court Standards for Guardianship, which were developed by the National College of Probate Judges and the National Center for State Courts.[6] Measures that states have taken reflect four trends (Quinn, 2005):

1. Enhanced, procedural due process safeguards including meaningful notice, representation by counsel, and the presence of alleged incapacitated persons at hearings
2. Functional determinations of incapacity, relying less on medical labels and more on evidence concerning how the person functions in society
3. Emphasis on less restrictive alternatives
4. Strengthening accountability of guardians, including better reporting requirements, training for guardians, court oversight, and meaningful notice

Specific examples of state initiatives include the following:

Δ *Arizona's Supreme Court oversees a certification program for all public and private guardians (National Association of State Units on Aging, 2006). A similar program will begin in Texas in September 2007.*

Δ *New York provides for the appointment of "special guardians for protective arrangements" who are appointed for a short period of time to perform specific tasks or transactions such as selling homes or spending down assets and applying for Medicaid (N.Y. Mental Hygiene Law § 81.16[b]).*

Δ *In New Jersey, if a hospital ethics or "prognosis committee" determines that a patient's prognosis is hopeless, a specially appointed guardian may be appointed who has the authority to withhold treatment. In the case of elderly residents in long-term care, the state Office of the Ombudsman must determine that the decision does not constitute abuse (Section 4: N.J.S.A.3B:12-4).*

Protective Custody

A few states have created special provisions for "protective custody" of people who are incapacitated or gravely disabled for reasons other than mental illness and who are at risk for abuse, neglect, or exploitation. Under these statutes, designated individuals may remove adults from their homes and place them in protective settings for short periods to assess their protective service needs. The goal is to remove the immediate risk, stabilize the situation, and determine whether the impairment is permanent or temporary. These statutes vary widely with respect to who can initiate placements and under what circumstances. Examples include the following:

Δ *In Texas, APS can place into protective custody elderly or disabled persons who are in need of protective services and lack the capacity to consent to them (Texas Human Resources Code § 48.208). The statute has been used effectively to meet the needs of people suffering from self-neglect.*

Δ *In Montana, APS workers who have reasonable grounds to believe that older persons or persons with developmental disabilities are being abused, neglected, or exploited may place them into protective custody (MCA 52-3-804 [5][b]). The placement can be maintained for two days during which services are provided or a petition for guardianship is filed. APS is the only entity that can provide protective custody.*

Δ *In Florida, vulnerable adults may be taken into protective custody under two circumstances, both of which require court orders: (1) vulnerable adults who lack capacity to consent to protective services can be taken into custody for a period of sixty days for further evaluation in determining their mental status; and (2) when a vulnerable adult who lacks capacity to consent is in imminent risk of death if protective measures are not taken. Removals require the collaboration and approval of law enforcement and medical personnel (Chapter 415, Florida Statutes).*

Δ *In Utah, unlike other states, there are circumstances in which it is possible to order protective custody for nonconsenting victims who have capacity but refuse to take steps to protect themselves. According to the statute, "a peace officer may remove and transport, or cause to have transported, a vulnerable adult to an appropriate medical or shelter facility if the officer has probable cause to believe that by reason of abuse, neglect, or exploitation there exist emergency exigent circumstances and (a) the vulnerable adult will suffer serious physical injury or death if not immediately placed in a safe environment; (b) the vulnerable adult refuses to consent, or lacks the capacity to consent; and (c) there is not time to notify interested parties or to apply for a warrant or other court order." The peace officer must notify APS of these actions within four hours. APS or the division must then file petitions with the court for emergency protective orders. APS may also obtain emergency orders for temporary protection of no more than three working days by contacting the local district attorney or the state attorney general. If a client lacks the capacity to consent, the worker obtains a letter from a physician or psychologist stating this and prepares an affidavit for the court (Utah Code § 62A-3-308).*

Special Challenges

States have enacted countless other measures to prevent elder abuse and respond to its effects. Although it is beyond the scope of this chapter to describe them all, several important trends and areas of activity are described.

Reducing Abuse of Powers of Attorney (POAs)

Many of the abuses associated with powers of attorney (POAs) and durable powers of attorney (DPAs) that were described in Chapter 5 can be attributed to the lack of safeguards and oversight. For example, few states require that POAs be recorded or registered, or that principals be notified when attorneys-in-fact use their powers. Many principals do not realize the extent of the authority they are assigning to others.

Chapter 5 also referred to the Uniform Durable Power of Attorney developed by the National Conference of Commissioners on Uniform State Laws (NCCUSL). NCCUSL is an organization of lawyers, judges, and law professors who are appointed to draft proposals for uniform and model laws. In 2006, NCCUSL revised its Uniform Durable Power of Attorney to add additional safeguards and remedies. The new model law, which contains a sample form, describes minimum fiduciary duties of agents, expressly states (rather than implies) gift-making authority, and revokes spouse-agents' authority in the event of divorce or annulment.[8] Another major change from the earlier version is that all POAs are durable (survive incapacity) unless they expressly indicate otherwise. This is in contrast to the earlier version that required special language stating that the powers were intended to be durable.

State initiatives to prevent abuse involving POAs include the following:

Δ *North Carolina requires that POAs and DPAs be recorded with registrars of deeds (N.C. Gen. Stat. § 32A-11).*
Δ *In Washington, principals, agents, or certain other interested individuals can ask courts to get involved when problems arise. Courts can order agents to give accountings to the principal or to a third*

party, interpret or modify the powers, decide whether a third person must honor a power of attorney, or remove the agent.[9]

Preventing Predatory Lending

Although anyone can fall prey to predatory lenders, elderly homeowners are believed to be at particularly high risk. According to the Center for Responsible Lending, twenty-four states have passed antipredatory lending laws.[10] Predatory practices that are addressed include *property flipping*, which is when first-time homebuyers are targeted by "flippers" who arrange loans on homes that they bought cheap, made only cosmetic repairs on, and sold at inflated prices. Consequently, buyers are left with loans for the inflated sales price. *Loan flipping* is when the broker encourages the homeowner to refinance several times over a short period to generate fees for the broker (thereby stripping the homeowner of equity). Predatory loans also typically have stiff prepayment penalties. Prepayment penalties occur when a buyer pays off a loan early. These penalties are usually based on a percentage of the outstanding balance at the time of prepayment or a specified number of months of interest. Borrowers with subprime loans often cannot afford the penalties when they need to refinance. According to a report on subprime lending by the HUD/Department of the Treasury Task Force, about 70% of subprime loans contain prepayment penalties, whereas only 1% to 2% of prime loans include prepayment penalties (Stein, 2001). Predatory lenders also trap seniors into *deed theft* scams, where the senior is asked to sign over the deed to their home in order to "refinance" it. The senior is then made a tenant in his or her own home and is quickly evicted.

North Carolina's predatory lending statute[11] is widely considered the gold standard. It prohibits predatory flipping, sets a threshold for lenders' fees for high-cost loans at 5%, and protects consumers from abusive practices related to late fees (e.g., declaring all payments subsequent to a late payment also late). A study of the North Carolina law showed that it resulted in a reduction of loans with predatory terms without restricting the access or increasing the cost of loans to borrowers with imperfect credit (U.S. House of Representatives, 2003).

Adapting Restraining Orders to Meet Elders' Need for Protection

As described in Chapter 5, restraining orders are an important protection for elderly victims. Some states have created new orders or added protections for elderly victims.

Δ *California's "elder or dependent adult abuse restraining order" can be used to protect people from abusive roommates, atten-*

*dants, and other nonrelatives as well as spouses, intimate part-
ners, and other family members. The orders are a protection
against physical and financial abuse, neglect, abandonment, and
treatment that results in physical harm or mental suffering.*[12]

Δ *Colorado has a restraining order that provides protection against
emotional abuse of the elderly (Colo. Rev. Stat. § 13-6-107).
The order may restrain a party from repeated acts that constitute verbal threats or assaults, or verbal harassment. The law
also addresses the inappropriate use of medications, physical or
chemical restraints, and powers of attorney.*

Δ *New York's "limited orders of protection" permit abusers to remain
in victims' homes under certain conditions (e.g., they do not use
drugs or alcohol). The order is particularly useful for elder abuse
victims who have mixed feelings about family abusers who have personal problems and with whom they do not want to sever ties.*[13]

Δ *In 2006, Maine, Vermont, and New York passed laws that allow
judges to include pets in protective orders. The laws were passed in
recognition of the fact that harming pets is a common tactic used
by domestic violence perpetrators and that battered women often
delay the decision to seek safety out of fear for their animals' welfare (Ascione & Arkow, 1999; McIntosh, 2002). One study showed
that over 71% of battered women reported that their batterers had
harmed, killed, or threatened animals (Ascione & Arkow, 1999).*

Preventing Abuse in Long-Term Care Facilities

Recognizing that regulation alone has not been effective in preventing abuse
and neglect in long-term care facilities (U.S. General Accounting Office,
1999, 2002), states have taken increasingly aggressive measures to remedy
the situation. Most states now have laws requiring criminal background
checks for current and prospective employees and forbid facilities from
hiring applicants who have been convicted of certain crimes. Generally,
those applicants who have committed "crimes against persons," sexual
crimes, and crimes having to do with families are disqualified. Applicants
may be permanently disqualified or prevented from working for specified
time periods (typically five or ten years). States may also direct agencies to
consider mitigating circumstances, such as employees' age at the time they
committed crimes or the length of time since the crimes.

Some states have encountered problems in implementing these laws.
For example, when Pennsylvania prohibited long-term care facilities from
hiring applicants with certain criminal convictions, the state's Supreme
Court held that some aspects of the law were unconstitutional (U.S.
Department of Health and Human Services, 2006). A pilot program by

the Centers for Medicare and Medicaid Services is exploring how states can perform affordable background checks and evaluating the effectiveness of checks.[14]

Other approaches to improving care in long-term care facilities include the following:

Δ *Arkansas enacted a law in 1999 that requires nursing homes to report all deaths to local coroners and gives county coroners legal access to conduct investigations in facilities following residents' deaths.[15] A study of death investigations by the National Institute of Justice is exploring the impact of the law on the quality of resident care in the state (Lindbloom et al., 2005).*

Δ *"Granny cams." Some states, including New Mexico and Texas, have passed laws that let families install surveillance cameras in nursing home residents' rooms. Other states have debated the approach, raising questions about how tapes that capture abuse should be handled (e.g., should facilities have access to them and can they be used as evidence in criminal or civil legal matters) (Moskowitz, 2003).*

Δ *Operation Guardian, a project of the California Attorney General's Office, conducts surprise inspections of skilled nursing facilities.[16] A group that includes district attorneys, city attorneys, fire marshals, building code inspectors, ombudsmen, health inspectors, and geriatric care specialists identifies violations of federal, state, and/or local laws and regulations.*

Δ *New York State's Public Health Law creates a private right of action for nursing home abuse. Any residential health care facility that injures a resident by virtue of violating any federal statute or code is liable. Some of the more common grounds for suing nursing homes include negligence, wrongful death, intentional tort, negligent hiring and supervision, and breach of statutory/regulatory rights, duties, or responsibilities.[17]*

Δ *After a* Chicago Sun-Times *investigation revealed that one hundred registered sex offenders and sixty-one parolees convicted of nonsex crimes were living in nursing homes statewide, Illinois became the first state to require state police criminal background checks on nursing home residents. The law, which was passed in 2006, requires the state's Department of Public Health to develop monitoring plans for residents identified as having violent and sex-related convictions. In addition, nursing homes must place sex offenders in private rooms and notify all residents when offenders are housed in the facility. Homes must also provide plans for resident safety and to notify residents of offenders' background.[18]*

Preventing Abuse by In-Home Helpers

Just as states are requiring criminal background checks for current and prospective employees in long-term care facilities, some are also exploring ways to improve the screening of in-home-care providers. Some states permit home-care agencies to access criminal records and have established criteria to disqualify workers.

However, some states have encountered problems in developing screening policies. Just as keeping dangerous workers out of the market is a problem, so too is keeping rehabilitated or nondangerous ex-offenders in. When New Jersey passed a law requiring all home-care workers to have FBI fingerprint checks, for example, they discovered that 400 current employees had committed disqualifying crimes (Layton, 2001). Many had been working for years, and losing them would have dealt a devastating blow to the system. The state was able to get some of the workers exempted. The need for research on which to base hiring decisions is described in Chapter 9.

WHAT TRIBES ARE DOING

In 2006, the National Congress of American Indians passed Resolution #SAC-06-073, "Developing a Comprehensive Tribal Response to Elder Abuse." In doing so, the Congress "endorsed and recognized the importance of taking a proactive stance toward identifying and responding to elder abuse." The resolution calls for the establishment of tribal laws and procedures, supports the development of professional and family training, and encourages collaboration among tribal nations, the federal government, tribal justice systems, and community agencies in providing needed services for victims and offenders living in tribal communities.

In 2002, the National Indian Council on Aging (NICOA) launched a project, funded by the National Center on Elder Abuse, to explore elder abuse in Indian country, including areas of need and promising responses. The initiative included a review of the literature, discussions with experts, a national survey of professionals, and focus groups (Nerenberg, Baldridge, & Benson, 2003).

Several overarching themes emerged. "Key informants," including researchers, service providers, and elders, called for prevention and intervention programs that draw from traditional Indian values and beliefs and that address social, economic, and historical factors that contribute to abuse and neglect. Specifically, they called for programs that do the following:

• Promote family unity and cooperation
• Reflect traditional models of dispute resolution

- Employ informal community networks
- Attempt to prevent abuse by maintaining or supporting families and preserving and restoring cultural values and traditions
- Address "structural" inequalities and antecedents that place elders at risk. This includes, for example, decreasing younger family members' dependence on elders through jobs that pay adequate salaries. Education and access to health care, daycare, and eldercare services are also viewed as critical. It was further noted that income maintenance programs must reflect the intergenerational structure of Indian families, recognizing that elders will spend income to care for children and grandchildren during hard times.

Key informants also emphasized the need for extensive planning to ensure that programs meet tribal needs and are supported by tribal leaders. The planning process itself needs to reflect traditional Indian approaches such as consensus-building and intergenerational dialogue. In addition, all programs need to be evaluated to make sure they accomplish their intended objectives.

Although tribal codes are seen as essential in providing authority to intervene and to establish the roles and responsibilities of tribal and nontribal agencies, codes alone were not viewed as a solution. In fact, codes that do not provide for services are perceived as harmful to families. It was also noted that codes should be designed to maintain family units whenever possible.

Key informants further identified challenges that tribes face, including (1) coordinating service delivery, (2) ensuring justice, (3) training professionals, and (4) meeting the demand for services. The following sections describe these challenges as well as programs and initiatives that have been crafted to address them.

Improving Coordination

Because tribal, federal, state, and county organizations may all be involved in investigating abuse and providing services, coordination can be challenging. For example, on reservations with more than one tribe, separate law enforcement or social service programs may need to work together, and on reservations that extend across state lines, multiple state and county personnel may be involved. Other entities that have a role to play include tribal court personnel, social service providers, and housing and health services providers.

Tribes have fostered coordination among tribal departments and nontribal entities through interagency agreements, task forces, and multidisciplinary teams and planning councils. Examples include the following:

Δ *The Standing Rock Reservation has a multidisciplinary team that includes representatives from several tribal Veterans Administration, Indian Health Service, and Bureau of Indian Affairs (BIA) programs. It is coordinated by the tribe's Community Health Representative (CHR) program. The team reviews cases and addresses problems with service coordination.*

Δ *The Blackfeet Tribe Elder Protection Team, a volunteer group, was created to review cases that are referred by family members or other concerned persons (the state of Montana does not provide or fund adult protective services on the reservation). The team includes representatives from BIA Social Services, Blackfeet Housing, Indian Health Services, a senior citizen center, and personal care providers.*

Δ *The Cherokee Nation's principal chief and tribal council have made it a priority to provide tribal services to elders. The Nation employs two full-time "Elder Advocates" to help elders access tribal services and, if needed, services outside the tribe. The advocates further help elders fill out applications, retrieve documents, and perform other tasks.*

Δ *The Pokagon Band of Potawatomi Indians is working with the Cass County (Michigan) Council on Aging and the Sheriff's Office to increase awareness about elder abuse. They are initially focusing on financial abuse under the guidance of the Pokagon Elders Council.*

Ensuring Justice

Civil or criminal courts at the federal, state, or tribal levels may have jurisdiction in abuse cases. Tribal elder abuse codes vary with respect to their coverage, what agencies are designated to respond, and what services are provided. Some tribes have developed elder abuse codes similar to state codes, whereas others have adapted codes to reflect traditional values and approaches to resolving conflicts. Traditional approaches are also being used in tribal courts.

Δ *The "Model Tribal Elder Protection Code," published in 1990 by the University of New Mexico's American Indian Law Center, contains provisions that tribes can adapt or modify and instructions to guide them. The code is a civil code designed to promote reporting and services to elders and their families.[19]*

Δ *The Navajo Nation passed an elder protection code in 1996. In 2002, the tribe began working with Three Ts Inc., a private nonprofit agency, to review the code and recommend changes. The* review included meeting with prosecutors, staff at senior centers, members of the Navajo Nation Bar Association, Indian Health Service representatives, and others. These activities revealed that those most likely to observe abuse were unfamiliar with the code, were unclear about the roles of various tribal agencies and departments in handling cases, and lacked the skills to handle complex situations. The findings and recommendations were presented to the Navajo Nation's Council on Aging and the Health and Social Services Committee (a standing legislative committee of the Navajo Nation Council).

Training Professionals

Professionals and nonprofessionals who work with abused and vulnerable Indian elders need tribe-specific information about the nature and extent of the problem. They also need information about elder abuse codes and their reporting responsibilities. Non-Indian professionals who work with Indian elders may perceive abuse and neglect differently from those they serve, and therefore, also need training. The following programs have addressed these needs:

Δ "Restoring the Sacred Circle: Responding to Elder Abuse in American Indian Communities" is a training video that was produced by the Oregon Department of Human Services (ODHS) in consultation with an advisory committee that included representatives from the Yakama Nation, Confederated Tribes of Warm Springs, Confederated Tribes of Grand Ronde, the Trenton Indian Service Area, the Nez Perce Tribe, the Quinault Indian Nation, Klamath Tribes, and the National Indian Council on Aging (NICOA). ODHS also produced a fourteen-minute video to be shown during "roll call" for tribal law enforcement. The video illustrates various types of abuse.[20]

Δ NECHI Training, Research and Health Promotions Institute of Edmonton, Alberta offers a course in elder abuse that covers the following topics:

  Δ The traditional role of elders within native culture
  Δ Four categories of elder abuse within the native community
  Δ Symptoms of abuse and neglect
  Δ Community resources
  Δ Factors that lead to abuse of the elderly
  Δ The ways in which grieving issues are linked to depression and/ or acting out behaviors in the elderly

The NECHI course also provides an opportunity for service providers to explore their feelings about working with elder abuse and to assess their strengths and weaknesses.

Δ *Project SHARE: Native American Elder Abuse Nurses' Training is a project of South Dakota State University's College of Nursing. It was designed to improve the health status of elderly Native Americans who experience a high rate of preventable acute and chronic illnesses. Developed in 2002 by Native American nurses and caregivers, the multimedia, culturally specific online continuing education program for nurses contains a section (Module 3)[21] that focuses on the following:*
  Δ *How changes in Native American culture have increased the risk for elder and substance abuse*
  Δ *Ways to work with Native American elders who are abused or have substance abuse problems*
  Δ *Identifying culturally appropriate nursing interventions for elders at risk for elder or substance abuse*

Meeting the Demand for Services

A major impediment to meeting the service needs of vulnerable Indian elders is a lack of adequate financial and human resources. "Mainstream" programs or services may be inaccessible, inappropriate, or unacceptable to vulnerable Indian elders as a result of the following:

- Age barriers. Some vulnerable elders may not be eligible for needed services as a result of age requirements. The qualifying age for some services, including those offered under Title VI of the Older American's Act, varies by tribe.
- Geographic barriers
- Language and literacy barriers. Some Indian elders do not speak English fluently, and some do not speak it at all.
- Distrust of, or nonresponsiveness by, non-Indian service agencies and law enforcement

Some tribes have attempted to address these limitations by improving access to mainstream programs. An example is the Cherokee Nation's "Elder Advocates" program, described earlier. Other tribes have developed new programs that better reflect the needs of Indian elders and their families. An example is the Jamestown S'Klallam's Family Group Conferencing program, which was described in Chapter 5. In addition, several tribes have developed culturally specific approaches to community awareness, which are described in Chapter 8.

CONCLUSIONS

Lack of federal guidance in shaping states' responses to elder abuse has had both positive and negative repercussions. On the positive side, it has spurred states to develop creative solutions to a wide range of highly complex and multifaceted challenges. In doing so, some states have probed new areas of public policy and fostered new relationships at the state and local levels. In some cases, states have built upon foundations laid by earlier advocacy movements. Policy makers and program developers have also watched what other states have done, refined and modified promising approaches, and ventured off in new directions. This experimental approach has yielded valuable insights and innovations.

On the other hand, this independence has also led to a lack of cohesion and wide variations across the country with respect to how abuse is defined and responded to. These include variations in what services and interventions are available and the number of cases that are reported, investigated, and substantiated. These differences have made it virtually impossible to develop a national profile of abuse or to anticipate national needs.

This chapter has merely scratched the surface in terms of what has been done. New state and tribal programs and policies are emerging on an almost daily basis. To take advantage of these innovations and the knowledge they have yielded, we need to create opportunities for states to learn from each other's experiences and explore how lessons learned in one state may apply to others. We also need to find ways to balance the benefits of states' and tribes' diversity with the need for cohesion and a national profile of elder abuse.

NOTES

1. For more information, see http://www.leg.state.vt.us/statutes/fullsection.cfm?Title=13&Chapter=167&Section=05363.
2. For more information, see http://www.miseniors.net/NR/rdonlyres/0E5BFE7E-BD49-4088-BF87-82A36BD83E11/0/ElderAbuseTFRecomm.pdf.
3. http://www.dhfs.state.wi.us/APS/index.htm.
4. Available online at http://www.courtinfo.ca.gov/forms/documents/gc335.pdf.
5. Beneficiaries' income is applied toward their care, with the state paying whatever portion of the actual costs the beneficiary's income cannot cover. Medicaid, however, allows patients to retain a portion of their income for approved services that are not covered by other third parties.
6. See http://www.ncpj.org/standard.html.
7. See http://www.abanet.org/aging/docs/guardian1.pdf.
8. The Uniform Durable Power of Attorney Act is available on the Web site of the National Conference of Commissioners on Uniform State Laws at http://www.nccusl.org.
9. See http://www.lawhelp.org/documents/1543119900EN.pdf? stateabbrev=/WA/.
10. See http://www.responsiblelending.org/issues/mortgage/reports/page.jsp?itemID=28546805.

11. See http://www.house.gov/htbin/leave_site?ln_url=http://www.kenan-flagler.unc.edu/assets/documents/CC_NC_Anti_Predatory_Law_Impact.pdf.

12. For more information on California's "elder or dependent adult abuse restraining order," see the Web site of the California Courts Self-Help Center at http://www.courtinfo.ca.gov/selfhelp/protection/eaproblems.htm

13. For more information on New York's "limited orders of protection," see http://72.14.253.104/search?q=cache:GtSfVLZf7-QJ:www.safehorizon.org/files/What_Expect_Crim_Crt_Bklt.pdf+New+York+%E2%80%9Climited+orders+of+protection%E2%80%9D&hl=en&ct=clnk&cd=4&gl=us.

14. For more on the CMS project, see http://www.cms.hhs.gov/SurveyCertificationGenInfo/Downloads/bc_GeneralInfo.pdf-.

15. P.L. 499, Arkansas Statutes [2005].

16. For more information on Project Guardian, see http://ag.ca.gov/bmfea/elder.php.

17. Can the law protect nursing home residents? (2006). Retrieved April 15, 2007, from http://www.ltccc.org/newsletter/documents/ltccc_fall2006_web.pdf.

18. For more on the Illinois law, see the Web site of A Perfect Cause at http://www.aperfectcause.com/artman/publish/article_2900.asp.

19. Information on the Model Tribal Elder Protection Code is available on the Web site of the American Indian Law Center at http://lawschool.unm.edu/ailc/publications.php.

20. Information on the videos is available on the ODHS Web site at http://www.oregon.gov/DHS/spwpd/abuse/videos.shtml.

21. The curriculum is available online at http://learn.sdstate.edu/share.

CHAPTER EIGHT

Community Outreach

INTRODUCTION

An essential element for preventing elder abuse is an informed public. This assumption has led abuse prevention groups at the local, state, tribal, national, and international levels to carry out community outreach campaigns. Yet, although the need for outreach is universally acknowledged, there is widespread disagreement about what outreach actually can or should attempt to accomplish. There are also wide variations in the approaches used, the audiences that are targeted, and the "messages" that campaigns convey.

This chapter describes these differences and provides examples. It begins by presenting some of the fundamental goals and assumptions behind outreach and describes how they shape specific campaigns. Several local, state, and national campaigns are described, as well as one tribal and one international campaign.

GOALS OF OUTREACH

The primary goals of most elder abuse outreach campaigns are to inform the public that help is available and to urge victims and witnesses to report. This is to ensure that those in need know that help is available and how to access it. But educating the public about abuse can also serve broader goals. It can shape public attitudes about the problem and what should be done about it, generate support for new or improved public policy, and enlist the public's help in stopping abuse. In addition, some campaigns have reinforced cultural traditions that hold elders in high esteem and affirmed families' responsibilities toward their elderly members.

Alerting Victims and Others That Help Is Available

Although public consciousness about abuse has clearly increased in the last two decades, many people are still unclear about what elder abuse is. Some believe that abuse only occurs in nursing homes or that the term only refers to physical violence against elders. Many victims and concerned third parties are unaware that help is available or how to access it. Many campaigns, therefore, describe the various forms of abuse and direct people to points of entry into the service delivery system such as APS programs or elder abuse help lines.

Because victims and others are likely to have apprehensions about disclosing abuse or about what will happen if they do, campaigns may further address these concerns. They may, for example, explain how the reporting system works and assure victims that their wishes, choices, and rights will be respected. Some campaigns address victims' denial, fear, or shame. They may attempt to motivate victims to seek help with messages like "You are not alone," or "Nobody deserves to be abused." Some, like the Texas Department of Protective and Regulatory Service's "Elder Abuse is Everybody's Business" campaign, which is described later in this chapter, negates the notion that abuse is a "family matter," and emphasizes instead that abuse is a community problem that calls for a concerned and vigilant public. Others, like California's "Face It—It's a Crime" campaign, also described later, emphasize the public's duty to hold perpetrators accountable. Some focus on specific forms of abuse. In recent years, for example, several communities have launched campaigns addressing telemarketing and mortgage fraud, and domestic violence.

Shaping Attitudes and Behavior

Many people have misconceptions or counterproductive attitudes about abuse or the response system. For instance, a number of people believe that certain types of abuse like investment or telemarketing fraud are the result of victims' gullibility or greed, and therefore, cannot be stopped. Other people believe that if they report abuse, it will have negative consequences for victims or their families, or that abusers will be treated unjustly. For these reasons, many campaigns have attempted to counter mistaken public attitudes. For example, campaigns that frame elder abuse as a crime or emphasize that it can happen to anybody remove the onus from victims and places it instead on offenders.

Negative attitudes about the elderly are believed by many to contribute to abuse. Some people believe that abuse is caused by the breakdown of cultural values and traditions. As a result, certain outreach campaigns have focused on instilling positive perceptions about the elderly, teaching children to respect elderly family members, and creating opportunities for intergenerational exchange (Podnieks & Baillie, 1995).

Using the media to change the public's attitudes and behaviors is sometimes referred to as "social marketing," an approach that has been used extensively in the field of public health. Social marketing employs many of the same techniques that commercial businesses use to persuade people to buy products or to change behaviors. These techniques include the use of commercials on television and radio, billboards, and ads in newspapers. Just as commercial marketers attempt to get the biggest "bang for the buck" by targeting advertising campaigns to groups that are most likely to buy products, social marketing campaigns target groups that are at heightened risk for problems. As described in Chapter 3, some advocacy groups have been extremely successful in using social marketing to change social norms. An example is Mothers Against Drunk Drivers (MADD), which has used the media to discourage people from driving while intoxicated. The results have been dramatic, with "designated driver" becoming part of our vocabulary and lifestyle. Family violence prevention advocates have also used the media effectively to radically alter public attitudes about appropriate behavior. Campaigns have conveyed the message that violence among family members is not acceptable and that society has a responsibility to stop it.

A few elder abuse outreach campaigns have targeted children. This approach is based on the assumption that preventing elder abuse requires changing attitudes instilled during childhood. The programs attempt to strengthen children's appreciation of older people, sensitize them to what it's like to be old, and enlist their help in reporting abuse.[1]

Shaping Public Policy

Public awareness campaigns can advance public policy objectives by helping the public understand problems and encouraging people to advocate for needed change. Campaigns can generate public debate as well as community support for specific policies. Family violence prevention advocates have, for example, generated support for public policy that criminalizes family violence. Some campaign planners have attempted to reach policy makers directly. For example, planners of California's "Face It—It's a Crime" campaign selected Sacramento, the state's capital, as one of its target counties so that state legislators would be sure to get the message.

Reaching Underserved Groups

Targeted outreach has been used to overcome geographic, functional, and cultural barriers that impede access to services and information.

Underserved groups that have been targeted for outreach include elders in long-term care facilities, homebound elders, and elders who are members of diverse cultural communities.

Reaching victims in long-term care facilities is extremely difficult because the facilities, which may be responsible for the abuse, have control over victims' access to information. In addition, many residents are likely to have physical or cognitive impairments that make it impossible for them to ask for help. A "code of silence" among workers purportedly discourages many who observe abuse by coworkers from reporting abuse. Reaching homebound elders entails many of the same problems. Perpetrators often control victims' access to the phone, e-mail, mail, or visitors. Extreme caution has to be taken when encouraging institutionalized or homebound victims to disclose abuse to avoid endangering them further.

One approach to reaching homebound or isolated seniors is to enlist the help of "gatekeepers." The term *gatekeeper* refers to individuals who have access to elders, including homebound or hard to reach groups. Gatekeepers include postal workers, employees of utilities companies, barbers, grocers, and clergy. There are many examples of successful elder abuse prevention gatekeeper programs listed on the "promising practices" section of the National Center on Elder Abuse's Web site.[2]

The obstacles that members of specific cultural communities face in accessing services, which include language and literacy barriers and fear of negative consequences, have already been described at length. Culturally specific outreach campaigns that target specific communities address these obstacles. These campaigns further acknowledge the important role that culture plays in how members of specific cultural communities experience and think about abuse and how it influences if, when, and to whom victims turn for help. Culturally specific campaigns have also reinforced cultural attitudes and values that support family cohesiveness. And finally, they have sensitized families, including children, to elderly members' needs.

THE IMPACT OF OUTREACH

Little is known about the impact of outreach, and the few existing studies have yielded puzzling findings. This lack of information about impact is troubling, as it threatens to discourage APS and other service providers from undertaking outreach for fear of generating more cases than they can handle.

This fear is not unfounded. Some communities have observed significant increases in reporting during or following outreach campaigns.

In the three months following the launch of California's "Face It—It's a Crime" campaign, which is described later, one county's APS program reported a 35% increase in reports.[3] Other communities and states, however, have reported only moderate increases in reports yielded by outreach campaigns or have noted that the number of reports levels off over time. These experiences reinforce the need for outreach campaigns to be monitored closely and for those carrying out campaigns to make sure that their communities are prepared to respond to a heightened demand.

One of the few efforts to explore the impact of outreach on elderly victims raised more questions than it answered (Davis & Medina-Ariza, 2001). Conducted by Victim Services, Inc. of New York, the study used a methodology developed in the field of domestic violence to analyze the impact of a twelve-month experimental outreach program. The program paired police officers with domestic violence counselors to respond to incidents of family violence in housing projects. Modeled after a campaign to prevent domestic violence, the program selected thirty housing projects to receive public education on elder abuse. Program staff: (1) held community meetings to discuss elder abuse; (2) placed posters in public areas of the housing projects; and (3) distributed leaflets, which included definitions of abuse, the legal rights of victims, and services available from the police and social service agencies.

The researchers also randomly selected households from participating and nonparticipating housing projects that reported elder abuse to the police. Counselors visited the elderly victims to discuss their legal options and service needs and encouraged them to report to the police if the abuse continued. When possible, the police spoke with abusers.

The impact of the outreach program was evaluated by checking police records for new incidents of abuse in the projects and interviewing victims six to twelve months following the incidents that had triggered the interventions. In doing so, they found that new incidents of abuse were more frequent among households that had received information. They also found a significant increase in reports of physical abuse, indicating that the interventions had not suppressed abuse and may have actually accelerated it.

These findings were in sharp contrast to those yielded by the earlier studies on domestic violence. The earlier studies had found that the outreach activities had resulted in significantly more reports to the police, which implied greater victim willingness to report, but the follow-up home visits did not reveal actual increases in violence in the families that had received education. In other words, the abusers were not incited to commit further violence after the intervention.

LOCAL, STATE, NATIONAL, TRIBAL, AND INTERNATIONAL CAMPAIGNS

Outreach campaigns have been carried out at the local, state, tribal, national, and international levels. The following examples describe general campaigns, gatekeeper programs, and culturally specific programs at these levels.

Local Outreach Campaigns

Outreach at the local level may be carried out by individual agencies or organizations, governmental entities, or coalitions. Local outreach programs offer several advantages. They can reflect communities' own populations and address their special needs, such as perceived or real barriers to access. They can also be very specific in describing services and resources (e.g., listing local agencies by name and providing phone numbers).

Local programs can also be monitored closely for impact, enabling those in charge to respond to changes in demand or to problems that arise. For example, if outreach activities generate a greater demand for services than local agencies can absorb, they can scale back outreach activities or advocate for more resources.

A disadvantage of local campaigns is that they are too expensive and labor intensive for many communities to carry out. In addition, many of the important avenues for communicating to the public—including newspapers, television, the Internet, radio, billboards, and other media—reach beyond the boundaries of a single city, county, or community.

Examples of single agency or local programs include the following:

Δ *Ventura County California's "Prescription for Prevention"* campaign was carried out by the county's district attorney to reach homebound seniors. The DA's office produced a one-page message on abuse and the office's services, which local pharmacists inserted in bags along with prescriptions. The same group developed a paper placemat with an elder abuse prevention message on it for home-delivered meal programs to distribute with meals.

Δ *Lakeshore Legal Aid* in Clinton Township, Michigan, provides advocacy for limited English proficiency and undocumented elderly victims of abuse, domestic violence, and sexual assault. The agency has conducted culturally appropriate and linguistically accessible outreach and community legal education on elder abuse.

Δ *WE ARE FAMILY: Outreach to African-American Seniors,* a program of the San Francisco Consortium for Elder Abuse

Prevention, was created in 1992 to raise awareness about elder abuse in the African American community (Nerenberg & Njeri, 1993). Concluding that outreach is most effective when it is personal, the "Leadership Group," which spearheaded the campaign, created opportunities for seniors and professionals to come together in an environment where the seniors felt comfortable asking for information and assistance. Churches and community centers hosted events that incorporated African American traditions and art forms—such as poetry, story telling, and music—into presentations about abuse and services. At these events, representatives from social service agencies and businesses that offer senior programs and discounts set up information tables and were available to talk to seniors informally. The Leadership Group also worked closely with trusted sources of information in the community, including clergy, civic organizations, community leaders, and the ethnic media. Another area of emphasis was ensuring that the agencies elders were referred to were prepared to respond appropriately and treated clients respectfully and in a timely manner.

State Outreach Campaigns

States have taken two primary approaches to outreach. Recognizing the benefits of engaging local communities in outreach campaigns, most states have chosen to support local efforts by providing communities with resources, technical assistance, and materials. They have, for example, hired advertising firms to plan campaigns and produce artwork and media placements that local communities can customize for their own use.

The economic advantages to this approach are obvious. Having a single entity conduct research and design materials is clearly more cost effective than having communities carry out these activities separately. The approach also results in a unified "look" and message within states.

In contrast, a few states have taken a second approach. These states operate statewide campaigns, in which state agencies carry out and control activities. The advantage of this approach is greater uniformity across the state. A disadvantage is that the approach does not reflect local variations in terms of their populations and resources. Examples of approaches to statewide campaigns are described below.

△ *The Texas Department of Protective and Regulatory Services (TDPRS) has, for many years, produced "Elder Abuse Prevention Kits" for its regional offices to use and share with other community groups. TDPRS works with a production company to produce the kits, which contain fact sheets, public service announcements (PSAs), camera-ready artwork, and other resources in both English and Spanish.[4] The Department also works with media outlets to disseminate information and produces novelty items like pens, magnets, magnifiers, and rulers that protective service staff can distribute at events for professionals and seniors.*

TDPRS has adopted different outreach messages over the years. The current campaign's message is "Protecting Vulnerable Adults from Abuse, Neglect, Financial Exploitation, or Isolation Is Everyone's Business," which encourages concerned citizens to get involved. A previous campaign, "Not Forgotten," focused on reducing isolation, a primary risk factor for abuse, and encouraged elders and dependent adults to stay active in their communities. Both campaigns emphasize that agencies alone can't protect the state's vulnerable citizens and enlist the community's help. To further promote this goal, TDPRS works with advisory boards and local citizens' groups to generate new resources. In addition, local community groups operate resource centers that provide food, supplies, and clothes to protective service clients; raise funds to make local shelters "elder-ready"; and sponsor caseworkers.

Δ   *"Elderly Pennsylvanians Deserve Honor and Respect," a culturally specific campaign that was carried out by the Pennsylvania Department of Aging in the mid-1990s, has served as a model for numerous other programs across the country. After observing that African American, Latino, and rural elders were less likely than other seniors to access services, the department contracted with an advertising agency to develop a campaign to reach these groups.*

Focus groups and individual interviews with seniors revealed that respect for elders remained high in the targeted communities. Elders also expressed a preference for campaigns that emphasized and reinforced honor and respect, as opposed to campaigns that focus on reporting abuse to authorities. On the other hand, professionals who were interviewed wanted a more hard-hitting campaign that emphasized reporting.

The Department chose to follow the seniors' recommendation and adopted the theme "Elderly Pennsylvanians Deserve Honor and Respect," which was used in brochures, posters, and radio and television PSAs. All of the materials depicted positive images of elders and caregivers. The primary targets of the campaign were elders, their families, neighbors, and anyone else who was likely to observe abuse. Like TDPRS, the Pennsylvania

Department of Aging developed the materials and encouraged local communities to customize them to reflect individual needs. The Department also provided communities with small grants to help them in this effort.

Δ *California's "Face It—It's a Crime" is an example of a campaign that was designed and carried out at the state level. The attorney general's office, which spearheaded the project, conducted interviews and focus groups with seniors and professionals before choosing its crime prevention message. The campaign targeted communities where awareness was low as reflected by low reporting rates and the findings of an "attitudes and awareness" survey (an exception was Sacramento County, which, as described earlier, was targeted to reach policy makers). Counties where awareness was lowest were given the highest priority and received the most resources, which included television commercials and PSAs, brochures, billboards, and flyers. The AG's office also hosted community forums and established a toll-free hotline to receive reports and requests for information generated by the campaign. The system directs callers to dial 911 in emergencies. In nonemergencies, callers who want to report abuse are directed to punch in their zip codes. They are then automatically transferred to their local APS units.*

Δ *Oregon's "Everyday Heroes" campaign acknowledges the important role of the public in abuse prevention. Each year, the Governor's Commission on Seniors honors members of the community who have recognized abuse and done something about it (e.g., investigated or reported to professionals). Professionals who have gone "above and beyond" the normal scope of their jobs may also qualify. The attorney general presents the reward at a ceremony.[5]*

Δ *Illinois' "Break the Silence Campaign" is sponsored by the state's Department on Aging. The campaign adopted July as Elder Abuse Awareness Month, and activities are carried out throughout the month. The state provides press releases, camera-ready artwork, and customized design services to communities that want to publicize the activities with billboards, advertisements, or other materials.*

National Outreach Campaigns

The national elder abuse outreach campaigns that have been carried out to date have focused on specific types of abuse and populations. An example of the former is AARP's campaign to raise awareness about telemarketing fraud. An example of the latter is a campaign conducted by the National Hispanic Council on Aging, which targeted Hispanic elders.

AARP's Anti–Telemarketing Fraud Campaign

When AARP became interested in telemarketing fraud, the organization conducted focus groups with its members to assess what they knew and thought about the problem. Among their important discoveries was that even though members felt that telemarketing fraud was wrong, they did not believe it was a crime. Many felt that when seniors got taken, it was their own fault, even when the perpetrators used deception or misrepresentation. In response, AARP launched a campaign that used the slogan "Telemarketing fraud is a crime. Report it." The focus of the campaign is obvious: to shift the blame from victims to perpetrators.

AARP also conducted research to learn more about victims (AARP, 1996). In doing so, they discovered that seniors who had already been taken by fraudulent telemarketers were highly likely to be defrauded again. Some were victimized repeatedly as they tried to recover what they had lost. AARP also discovered that telemarketers specifically target those who have victimized in the past, using "mooch lists."[6]

Drawing from these findings, AARP devised a campaign that targeted seniors who had previously been victimized. Working with the National Association of Attorneys General, they sponsored a "reverse boiler room" in which AARP volunteers, attorneys general, and representatives from other federal agencies contacted seniors whose names appeared on mooch lists confiscated in criminal investigations. The seniors were warned that they had been targeted by criminals and were provided with information to help them resist further abuse. The event has been replicated in communities across the country, and, as indicated in Chapter 4, several groups carried the idea further, operating reverse boiler rooms on an ongoing basis.

National Hispanic Council on Aging

The National Hispanic Council on Aging (NHCOA), a "network of networks" with chapters and affiliates across the country, has conducted two culturally specific outreach campaigns to raise awareness about elder abuse among Hispanics (Nerenberg, 2001).

The first campaign, launched in 1994 in Washington, D.C., focused on the obstacles that elderly Latina victims of domestic violence face in getting help. Among these obstacles are cultural taboos and fears about legal repercussions for reporting. A community board comprising representatives from social, legal, and health services was organized to identify community needs and appropriate services. An advisory group, most of whose members were elderly Nicaraguan and Salvadorian women who had come to the States during the civil wars in their countries, provided input.

Drawing from the groups' recommendations, NHCOA developed a program that enlisted the support of local organizations, businesses, churches, and families in raising awareness. Among the activities they sponsored were support circles to raise awareness and discuss abuse. The groups were made up of at least twenty-five elder members and were facilitated by advocates. Other activities included an awareness campaign in conjunction with the Spanish media. NHCOA also produced a video that depicts the lives of four elderly women, emphasizing their struggles both in their homeland and in the United States. The video, which also highlights the strengths of the women in overcoming their obstacles, was distributed to churches and schools. Intergenerational events were also conducted, during which speakers emphasized the community's respect for elders while also raising the issue of domestic violence (Nerenberg, 2001).

In a subsequent campaign, NHCOA helped local affiliates raise awareness about financial abuse. Among the challenges they addressed were seniors' reluctance to report abuse to law enforcement or to ask abusive adult children to move out of their homes because of their strong commitment to preserving families. Other challenges that were addressed were problems with access to services, which included the lack of service providers who speak Spanish and agency biases against helping immigrants. Also addressed were widespread health problems, which both increase elders' vulnerability to abuse and prevent them from accessing services.

To overcome these obstacles, NHCOA emphasized preventative approaches to reduce the risk of financial abuse and encouraged families to get involved. For example, the campaign encouraged trustworthy family members to assist elders who needed help cashing checks or transacting business. In addition, rather than addressing elder abuse as a separate issue, information about the problem was incorporated into health education materials and presentations. NHCOA also attempted to get churches involved, with mixed results. Although some churches were willing to disseminate information in church publications and to provide space for events, others shied away from getting involved in a "social issue."

Tribal Outreach Campaigns

The literature on abuse in Indian country has identified a variety of obstacles to raising awareness about abuse (Nerenberg, Baldridge, & Benson, 2003). These include the fact that Indian elders' perceptions about what is abusive conduct and how it should be handled may differ from those of non-Indians, younger family members, or professionals.

Financial constraints also prevent many tribes from producing costly materials like PSAs. In addition, some seniors lack access to services including transportation. In some remote areas, elders may not even have access to telephones. And, as described in the last chapter, a recurrent theme in the literature on abuse in Indian country is a preference for programs that build upon and reinforce traditional values and beliefs as a way of preventing abuse.

For these reasons, mainstream approaches to raising community awareness about elder abuse may not be effective or appropriate in Indian country. Some have observed that although it is important to provide information about reporting laws and tribal codes, this should not be the only emphasis of campaigns (Nerenberg, Baldridge, & Benson, 2003). Alternatives that have been suggested include campaigns that acknowledge and reinforce elders' role in traditional society and that sensitize youth about what it is like to be old and vice versa (sensitize elders about what it is like to be young today). Others have suggested the need for community conversations to explore how elders feel about abuse and what should be done about it.

- *The Great Lakes Inter-Tribal Council conducted an early public awareness and education campaign in the mid-1980s that provided direction for later campaigns[7] (Great Lakes Inter-Tribal Council, 1988). The campaign focused on acknowledging elders' contributions to their tribes. Children learned about their grandparents, made posters to honor them, and were sensitized about their needs. Other activities included a senior recognition event. Awareness activities were even conducted in detention centers. Outreach materials, including an outreach guide, were also produced.*

An International Campaign

On June 15, 2006, the International Network for the Prevention of Elder Abuse (INPEA) sponsored the first World Elder Abuse Awareness Day. Advocates gathered at the United Nations; and governments, NGOs, educational institutions, and religious groups sponsored educational programs, press conferences, and awareness events. The latter ranged from balloon races in the UK, to quilt-making in Canada, to theatrical performances. Events were held in Uganda, Sweden, Gambia, Nigeria, Israel, Albania, Korea, Ireland, India, and Cameroon, the United States, and Canada. A second annual event was held on June 15, 2007. INPEA produced the *Community Guide to Raise World Awareness on Adult Abuse Tool Kit* to help those who want to plan events.[8] The kit contains ideas, resources, and sample materials like proclamations and press releases.

CONCLUSIONS

Educating the public about a problem as complex and multidimensional as elder abuse is not easy. It is rendered even more challenging by the fact that many people hold preconceived notions and mistaken assumptions about the problem itself and how the response system operates. Further complicating matters is the fact that communities across the country define abuse in different terms and have response systems that operate differently. Our lack of knowledge about the impact of campaigns makes it impossible to anticipate the demand for services that campaigns will generate; and, because the response systems vary, we cannot assure victims about what to expect. And finally, our ability to mobilize communities to affect social change is limited by the fact that our field lacks a clear vision and consensus about the direction we need to take to achieve greater protection, justice, and safety for elders.

Despite these obstacles and limitations, we have made significant strides in educating the public about elder abuse, directing victims to needed services, and encouraging concerned citizens to get involved. The challenge today is to build on our experiences and successes so we can reach more elders. To do so effectively and responsibly, we need to have a common vision and dependable responses. The specific factors that need to be considered in order to do this are described in the next chapter.

NOTES

1. For more on outreach to children, see http://www.ncea.aoa.gov/NCEAroot/Main_Site/ Resources/Community_Outreach/Outreach_Kit/Chapter4/Ch4_3.aspx.
2. See http://www.ncea.aoa.gov/NCEAroot/Main_Site/Resources/Promising_Practices/PP_ Home.aspx.
3. For more on "Face It—It's a Crime", see http://www.ncea.aoa.gov/NCEAroot/Main_Site/ Resources/Community_Outreach/Outreach_Kit/Chapter4/Ch4_1_a.aspx.
4. The kits are available on TDPRS' Web site at http://www.dfps.state.tx.us/everyones business.default.asp.
5. http://www.oregoneverydayheroes.org.
6. For more on telemarketing fraud and victims' characteristics, see Chapters 2 and 4.
7. For more information about the campaign, see "Effective public awareness efforts in tribal communities," by the Great Lakes Inter-Tribal Council. The guide was prepared in 1988 pursuant to U.S. Dept. of Health and Human Services Administration on Aging, Grant No. 90AM0215 and is available from the Clearinghouse on Abuse and Neglect (CANE) at http://www.ncea.aoa.gov/NCEAroot/Main_Site/Library/CANE/CANE.aspx.
8. Available on INPEA's Web site at http://www.inpea.net/downloads/community_guide_1- 20-06.pdf.

CHAPTER NINE

Responding to Challenges

INTRODUCTION

Ensuring that elders have the services and protections they need is complicated by myriad new developments and challenges, many of which have been described in previous chapters. Our swelling elderly population demands that we fortify the safety net of protective, supportive, and legal services. The presence of increasingly frail elders in our communities requires heightened vigilance and new approaches to ensuring access to services. In the new environment of "consumer choice," we need to make sure that the long-term care "market" operates effectively and provides a sufficiently large and varied continuum of services to meet the diverse needs of frail "consumers." Our ever more diverse elderly population requires that we remove language and cultural barriers to services and acknowledge the special needs of communities whose experiences and values do not conform to those of the mainstream. Ensuring that we have a highly trained and vigilant professional workforce has become more difficult as the cases we're seeing become increasingly more complex and varied.

Our ability to meet these challenges is hindered by persistent and formidable obstacles. Foremost among these, perhaps, is our inability to agree on such basic issues as what elder abuse is and whom we should serve. Members of our network differ in our outlooks and ideologies. There are still glaring gaps in our understanding of elder abuse and in the effectiveness of services and interventions. And finally, as public awareness about elder abuse grows, our service delivery network has come under greater scrutiny. In some cases, the harsh criticism leveled against us suggests that the principles and values that have guided our work, including our prioritizing of freedom over safety in some situations, may not be understood or shared by the public.

This chapter discusses some of these challenges. It is not exhaustive. Other professionals and organizations have also compiled lists of unmet needs for services, training, advocacy, and research. I have not attempted to incorporate their work but rather, have presented areas of need that I believe have not received the attention they deserve. The chapter sets the stage for the final chapter, which proposes a plan for the future.

DEFINING ABUSE

Ironically, after more than a quarter century since our field's start, defining abuse still remains a primary challenge. The lack of consensus and clarity about the parameters and key features of abuse have stymied research, advocacy, and service development. As new opportunities present themselves to affect comprehensive public policy, our lack of agreed-upon definitions seriously impedes our ability to propose coherent and cohesive policy. Without common definitions, it is impossible to estimate the extent of the problem, service needs, and the costs of implementing programs.

It may never be possible to develop a single, universal definition of elder abuse and neglect. Definitions have to reflect their intended purposes, which vary widely. It is possible, however, to shed light on the impact and implications that various definitions have for practice. Questions that need to be considered include the following:

- Do we define victims based on their age alone, disability alone, or both?
- In defining perpetrators, do we focus on persons in positions of trust and confidence, or do we include strangers?
- How do we define "persons in positions of trust and confidence"? How do we define "strangers" in light of the fact that predators actively seek out victims and cultivate trust and confidence in order to abuse?
- How do we define caregivers and the "duty to provide care"?
- In defining abuse
  - Do we include unintentional or reckless acts, or only willful, malevolent ones?
  - Do we focus on conduct or its impact?
  - How do we measure abusive conduct and the harm it causes (what thresholds of frequency and lethality do we use)?

The definitions we use in different situations and settings have to reflect the repercussions or "stakes" involved in labeling abusers or abusive conduct. For example, definitions that are used to qualify victims or vulnerable elders for services will differ from those used to trigger sanctions for abusers. When the goal is to capture early-stage abuse or high-risk situations, broad definitions may be appropriate. However, when the goal is to punish offenders, narrower definitions are needed to capture the most serious and repeat offenders. A single agency may define abuse differently for different purposes.

Definitions may serve to do the following:

- Target high-risk groups for outreach or preventative interventions
- Determine whether elders are eligible for social or protective services
- Trigger abuse investigations
- Trigger sanctions for abusers (e.g., placing their names on abuse registries or initiating legal action)

Agencies, program developers, advocates, and policy makers also need to decide if and when it is appropriate and advisable to include *self-neglect* and *elder domestic violence* in definitions of elder abuse. The benefits and potential consequences of doing so were presented in Chapter 2.

I have repeatedly urged those who work with victims and abusers to join the definitional debates. Their input will help policy makers, researchers, and program developers anticipate what repercussions various definitions will have for practice. The outcome of these deliberations will directly affect practitioners' work.

There is obviously a tremendous amount of work that our field needs to undertake to define elder abuse and understand the implications of various definitions. Some of the specific information that is needed to inform this work will be discussed in more detail later in this chapter.

RESPONDING TO A MULTICULTURAL SOCIETY

The elderly population is becoming progressively multicultural, a trend that is expected to continue and intensify for the next two decades. By 2030, the older minority American population is projected to increase by 217%, compared to an 81% increase for the older white population (United States Department of Health and Human Services, Administration on Aging, 2006).

What impact will this have on practice? A great deal, as culture plays a prominent role in the types of abuse that occur and how abuse is perceived and responded to. Culture further affects attitudes about accepting services and shapes preferences with respect to services.

The literature on cultural issues in elder abuse has consistently called for alternatives to "one-size-fits-all" approaches. Instead, it calls for programs that reflect users' needs, experiences, values, and preferences. In developing culturally specific programs, we need to look at the historical, economic, and social factors that erode family support networks and create intergenerational strife. The literature has further called for holistic approaches that focus on whole families and communities, and the context in which abuse and neglect occur. For example, the heightened demands on caregivers that have resulted from intergenerational caregiving and kinship care in some communities have been frequently noted (Benton, 1998; Nerenberg, Baldridge, & Benson, 2003; Nerenberg & Njeri, 1993; Pinquart & Sörensen, 2005). Researchers and practitioners have further acknowledged the negative experiences that some members of minorities have had with the American criminal justice and social service systems and the impact of these experiences on their willingness to report abuse. In the case of immigrants, some have had negative experiences in their countries of origin, which continue to affect their decisions about seeking out and accepting help (Shipler, Anand, & Hadi, 1998).

Some of the emerging trends and developments in the field of elder abuse prevention may potentially have negative consequences for members of specific groups, which need to be explored. For example, studies of domestic violence have suggested that mandatory arrest policies have resulted in inappropriate arrests of poor women, women of color, and undocumented immigrant women (Harrison & Karberg, 2003). The extent to which these consequences may affect older victims is not yet known. But as domestic violence against elderly women is increasingly being recognized and domestic violence laws are being applied, we need to be aware of possible negative consequences. And, although programs that enable elders to use public funds to hire family members as caregivers may ease the intense strains that many minority caregivers experience, laws that disqualify caregivers who have criminal histories may disproportionately impact communities that are overrepresented in the criminal justice system.

DEFINING CAPACITY FOR SPECIFIC TASKS

Significant strides have been made in understanding cognitive deficits and their impact on elder abuse and its prevention. However, as new forms of abuse are identified and new interventions are explored, it has raised new questions about how to define and evaluate capacity with respect to the risk of abuse, service needs, and decision-making capacity. Specific areas of need include the following:

- Defining capacity in assessing abuse: Inducing incapacitated elders to execute or consent to certain actions or transactions may constitute abuse. However, there is a lack of consensus with respect to how capacity should be defined for certain actions such as giving gifts, getting married, consenting to sexual relations, or executing certain legal or financial transactions.
- Defining capacity to consent to or refuse services: Experts disagree about the criteria that should be used to determine when vulnerable elders have sufficient capacity to stop investigations and refuse specific services. They also disagree about when involuntary interventions or surrogate decision makers are needed.
- Defining capacity to participate in research (see Challenges to Research).

SERVICE NEEDS

Despite the rapid proliferation of new services and interventions, few, if any, communities have an adequate supply. Among the most commonly cited shortages are APS, guardians for elders with limited assets (including public guardians), and emergency services. Other critical needs that have received less attention are described below.

Services for Victims of Financial Crimes and Abuse

The devastating impact of financial abuse and crimes against elders has been frequently noted (Deem, 2000; Deem, Nerenberg, & Titus, 2007; Hafemeister, 2003; Rabiner, O'Keeffe, & Brown, 2006). Victims have lost homes and life savings; gone into debt; and suffered mental health problems, including substance abuse and depression. Few services, however, are available to help victims reduce their risk, recover assets, or treat trauma. This lack of services has been attributed by some to a pervasive attitude that financial crimes and abuse are less serious than physical abuse (Deem, 2000; Deem, Nerenberg, & Titus, 2007). This bias is apparent in the fact that most programs funded under the Victims of Crime Act are for victims of violence. APS programs and legal service providers for the elderly are likely to serve victims of some forms of financial abuse but not others. Few, for example, serve victims of telemarketing and investment fraud or identity theft.

Although the potential of daily money management (DMM) to reduce the risk of abuse has long been acknowledged, social service agencies have traditionally been reluctant to provide the service. This is a result of multiple difficulties, which include obtaining insurance for workers and volunteers and concerns about liability (American Association of Retired Persons, 1996; Nerenberg, 2003; Sacks, 1994; Wilber, 1995). Fortunately, technical assistance is increasingly becoming available to help agencies that wish to implement programs. A leader in this area is the Brookdale Center on Aging's Sadin Institute on Law, which operates the Money Management Assistance Program as part of its Reingold Elder Abuse Project. The program's goal is to encourage and assist care management agencies to safely and effectively offer DMM. The center has worked with senior centers, neighborhood social service agencies, senior housing complexes, and home-care agencies to help set up DMM programs. It provides technical assistance in program start-up, policy and procedures, risk management, documentation, and standardized forms.[1]

Other services that victims of financial abuse and crimes, and those at risk, may need include the following:

- Court advocacy
- Restitution advocacy and assistance filing for victim compensation
- Counseling, support groups, or coaching to help victims overcome the trauma of financial abuse and resist the advances of financial predators
- Capacity and undue influence assessments
- Private investigators or asset investigators to track down offenders and stolen assets
- Crisis intervention, including emergency shelter for those who have lost homes or been evicted from apartments, emergency funds for food and other basic necessities, and crisis counseling
- Support services, including help setting up new bank accounts, finding alternative housing (for those who have lost homes as a result of abuse), addressing problems with creditors, finding trustworthy attendants, and applying for public benefits
- Legal assistance to void contracts, recover misappropriated assets and property, and annul bogus marriages or adult adoptions. In particularly short supply are legal services to address new and increasingly complex forms of financial abuse including predatory lending, identity theft, and mass-marketing fraud. Victims of identity theft, for example, may need help defending themselves against criminal charges for crimes committed by others in their names or if they are held responsible for depositing and drawing on bad checks sent to them as sweepstakes prizes.

Services for Abused or Vulnerable Elders with Dementias and Mental Illnesses

The need for services and interventions for elders with diminished capacity or mental illnesses is becoming particularly critical and will continue to grow as more frail individuals live in the community. Those who lack family, friends, and surrogates (sometimes referred to as "unbefriended elders") are particularly vulnerable.

APS workers and others are likely to discover confused, disoriented, or delusional elders in severely deteriorated conditions or settings. Often, it is unclear whether their impairments are permanent or the result of treatable, reversible conditions. As described in Chapter 5, hospitalization may be needed to evaluate their conditions or help them recuperate. In some instances, APS can work with police and mental health professionals to arrange for hospitalizations under "mental health holds," during which, patients' need for mental health treatment is assessed. But because dementia is not considered to be a mental illness, these laws typically do not cover elders with dementias. Some states, however, have expanded their mental health laws to extend coverage to persons with dementias. Others have developed special "protective custody laws," which are similar to mental health holds in that they allow police or others to hospitalize severely incapacitated people. Rather than assessing clients' need for psychiatric treatment, the goal of protective custody is to assess their need for protective services. Despite these initiatives, meeting the needs of confused, disoriented, or delusional elders in severely deteriorated conditions or settings remains a serious problem for APS and other workers.

Also lacking are surrogate decision makers for elders with dementias and mental illnesses who have not designated surrogates or executed advance directives prior to the onset of incapacity. These individuals may need others to act on their behalf, protect their interests, conduct business for them, or make decisions about their care. Options include representative payeeship, guardianship, and surrogate medical decision makers. These options are in short supply in many communities, particularly for elders with limited assets.

Many advocates consider guardianship to be the option of last resort when less restrictive alternatives are lacking or have been exhausted. In reality, however, few alternatives exist for people once they have lost capacity (many options, including trusts and powers of attorney, must be executed prior to the onset of incapacity). A group of professionals in San Francisco identified the following situations in which the need for less restrictive alternatives warrant exploration (Quinn & Nerenberg, 2005):

- When authority is needed to make single or limited medical treatment decisions
- When authority is needed to authorize placement in long-term care facilities
- When authority is needed to make financial or legal transactions on a limited or one-time-only basis (e.g., freeze assets to stop exploitation)
- When authority is needed to assess the capacity and protective service needs of elders who are gravely disabled or at imminent risk

The San Francisco group also researched what other communities are doing to meet these needs. Among the options they looked at were "limited guardianship" (guardianship that is limited in scope or duration), statutes or court processes for requesting authority to make decisions in specific instances (e.g., for single medical or placement decisions), and the use of ethics committees to provide guidance to surrogate decision makers or to actually serve as surrogates (Karp & Wood, 2003; Quinn & Nerenberg, 2005).

As more frail elders hire and supervise their own home-care workers, those with diminished mental capacity will undoubtedly need help. The extent to which abused elders with cognitive impairments need and can benefit from other protective services and interventions, including shelters, safety planning, and counseling, has not yet been determined.

Services for Perpetrators and Those at Risk of Abusing

Perpetrators of elder abuse and neglect span the spectrum from exhausted, overburdened caregivers to predators who prey on vulnerable elders to support lavish lifestyles. Consequently, interventions for perpetrators, their families, and those at risk of abusing also span a broad spectrum. Among the most critical gaps are services for caregivers, services for perpetrators with mental illnesses and dementias, services for the families of perpetrators with mental illnesses or dementias, and services for perpetrators of domestic violence.

Services for Caregivers at Risk of Abusing

Many communities have a wide range of resources available for family caregivers, including respite, support groups, and educational programs. The extent to which these services reduce the risk of abuse and neglect has not yet been explored. And, although researchers have made important discoveries about the risk factors associated with abuse by caregivers, this knowledge has yet to be translated into practice. These risk factors—which include poor premorbid relationships between caregivers and patients, caregivers' fears about abusing, and aggression by patients—have not, for example, been included in screening tools for dementia care programs or APS programs. Nor have they been included in "self-assessment tools" to help caregivers identify red flags. Counseling and education programs for caregivers also need to be adapted to reflect new knowledge as it becomes available.

Services to help caregiving families resolve conflicts or to help caregivers address conflicts with those they care for are also needed. The promising results that caregiver mediation and conferencing programs have started to yield suggest that these new paths should be explored further.

Elders and their caregivers also stand to benefit from education and support to help them carry out their roles as "long-term care consumers." This includes assistance in deciding when services are needed and how to select and monitor providers and facilities. Elders and their families can also benefit from tips to avoid abuse such as requiring receipts for purchases made by helpers, employing more than one worker (with alternating shifts), closely monitoring bank accounts and phone bills, keeping important financial information and documents locked up, and making or arranging for unannounced visits to check on elders' care.

Services for Perpetrators with Mental Illnesses and Dementias

Many communities have critical shortages of mental health services, which can be traced back to the movement to deinstitutionalize the chronically mentally ill that began during the 1970s. The plan to replace hospitals with community mental health services—including halfway houses, case management, and crisis clinics—was never fully implemented, and some components of the plan were later eliminated, resulting in many chronically mentally ill people being left homeless or living in cheap housing with little or no supervision.

As a result of these shortages, parents often choose or are pressured to care for their own mentally ill children. Adult children with mental illnesses may be abusive or become abusive when they stop taking medications. Although, in these situations, police and others have the authority to take the abusive person into involuntary custody and assess their need for psychiatric treatment, the laws typically allow for a maximum of three days of involuntary placement. During that time, individuals often become stable and are then released back to their homes. However, some quickly go off their medications again and the cycle of violence continues. As the parents of these children age, they may become less able to protect themselves.

When mentally ill abusers become involved in the criminal justice system, both they and their victims are likely to need advocates. Elderly parents who are assaulted by their adult children often want to see their children helped and, therefore, refuse to press charges even when they have been seriously injured. In addition, defense attorneys may try to intimidate or scare the parents into recanting their statements by saying their sons or daughters may face lengthy prison sentences (Stein, 2003). Advocates are needed to help these parents understand their options and explore alternatives.

Mentally ill perpetrators also need advocacy services to ensure that they are treated fairly and appropriately. Appropriate interventions may include being ordered to undergo psychiatric care and agree to medication through sentencing, probation, and parole terms. Other interventions and services that may be needed include long and short-term hospitalization, mental health case management, crisis intervention, and medication monitoring.

Abusers with Alzheimer's disease or other dementias are also increasingly getting entangled with law enforcement and have received little attention (Stein, 2003). They too can benefit from advocacy to ensure that they are treated appropriately and humanely. When police are summoned for domestic disturbances, they may not realize that violent partners have dementias, or they may make arrests anyway to comply with domestic violence laws. As a result, perpetrators with dementias may be jailed for hours or even days. Complicating matters further is the fact that dementias are often progressive, and determining when people are no longer culpable for their actions is not easy. People with early-stage or mild dementias may still understand the nature of their actions and should, therefore, be held accountable. However, the point at which they can no longer be held responsible may be difficult to determine. In addition, careful assessments are needed to determine whether aggressive or violent behavior can be controlled through medication or by other means, and when placement in secured facilities is required.

Services for Family Members of Perpetrators with Mental Illnesses and Dementias

Families of abusers with mental illnesses or dementias may also need services and information. This includes instruction in how to avoid abuse, protect themselves, see to it that their loved ones get appropriate help, remove or secure weapons, and manage difficult behaviors. Those whose family members become involved in the criminal justice system are likely to need education about the system and coaching to help them become effective advocates. The National Alliance for the Mentally Ill, a national organization for the families of people with mental illnesses, offers information about how to advocate for family members in the criminal justice system. The program, which has local branches around the country, is not, however, geared for the elderly.

Services for Perpetrators of Domestic Violence

Few communities have services to help perpetrators of domestic violence acquire new insights or skills, or to make amends to their victims or communities. This includes voluntary or court-ordered treatment programs. In particularly short supply are programs for women and nonintimate partners. Existing services were described in Chapter 5.

Housing and Shelter

The serious shortage of low-income or subsidized housing for the elderly that exists in many communities is a serious obstacle for many victims. The need for housing is particularly great in rural areas. Some communities have responded by working with Housing and Urban Development (HUD) officials to give abused or vulnerable elders priority for subsidized housing or arranging for "transitional housing" while they look for new, permanent housing.

Despite progress in this area (see Chapter 5), most communities still lack shelters for elderly victims. In particular, shelters are needed that can accommodate residents with physical and cognitive impairments, men, or victims of nonviolent crimes such as neglect and financial abuse.

MEETING THE CHALLENGE OF "CONSUMER CHOICE"

As "consumer choice" programs proliferate, we need to determine how frail elders are faring in the "long-term care marketplace" and how consumer choice programs impact the risk of elder abuse and the need for protective and supportive services. To do so, we must first consider some assumptions behind the consumer choice model.

For markets to operate effectively, certain conditions must be met:

- Consumers must have an adequate supply of products or services to choose from.
- They must have adequate information about those products and services.
- They must be capable of exercising choice (they must have decision-making capacity and be free from coercion or undue influence).
- They must have recourse when things go wrong.

At present, these conditions are not adequately being met. Most communities have severe shortages of in-home helpers, a mainstay of community-based long-term care and consumer choice programs. Critical information about helpers, including their criminal backgrounds, is often not available. In addition, there has been little discussion about how to evaluate elderly consumers' ability to make decisions about their care. And finally, the extent to which the protective service network is prepared to respond when things go wrong is not known.

The shortage of home-care workers stems from the low pay workers receive and the lack of basic benefits and protections they receive. As a result, consumers are being forced to "make do" and take such risks as hiring caregivers with criminal records, a situation that is getting worse (Nerenberg, 2002a; USGAO, 1996).

Clearly, the rising number of in-home helpers with criminal histories suggests that consumers need information about their prospective employees' criminal histories. However, few states permit individual consumers to access information about prospective employees' criminal backgrounds and in states that do, the information is likely to be incomplete. For example, criminal records do not contain information about charges that are eliminated under plea negotiations. In addition, state records do not contain information about crimes committed in other states, which is a problem because many predators travel from state to state.

The shortage of workers and lack of monitoring has become so serious that in some communities, probation and parole officers are purportedly encouraging those they supervise to become helpers. Reports of workers using other people's identities to get jobs are also becoming increasingly common.

Proponents of consumer choice contend that most elders, even those with moderate dementias, are capable of making basic decisions about the caregivers they want to hire (Squillace & Firman, 2004). These advocates, however, fail to differentiate between elders who have trusted friends or family members they want to hire, and those who must find, screen, and supervise strangers. The latter case clearly requires significantly more complex intellectual skills, and there has been little discussion about how capacity to perform these tasks should be defined or measured. There has also been little discussion about the skills that elders need to protect themselves against abuse by caregivers, which may include detecting theft, confronting abusers, withstanding undue influence, negotiating conflicts, and seeking help.

Although some consumer choice advocates concede that not all elderly consumers can protect themselves, they argue that the traditional safety net of protective services offers recourse when problems arise (Matthias & Benjamin, 2003; Squillace & Firman, 2004). In practice, however, APS and other agencies face obstacles in helping clients who have independently hired abusive caregivers. Investigating and proving abuse is complicated by multiple factors, including the fact that there are seldom witnesses; victims are extremely vulnerable to retaliation, coercion, or undue influence; victims may not understand that they have been abused (particularly when the abuse is financial); and many victims want to protect their abusers. Agencies that oversee programs have also been reluctant to get involved against the wishes of elderly employers, or they have been prevented from doing so, even when there have been allegations of abuse.

A few initiatives have been undertaken to address the shortage of in-home workers and screen out workers who pose a risk. To increase the supply of caregivers, advocates have worked with unions and programs for displaced workers (those who have lost jobs as a result of downsizing or other economic conditions and people returning to the workforce after extended absences) (Nerenberg, 2002). The Home Care Aide Association of America has attempted to achieve greater accountability by proposing a uniform classification system that reflects workers' training, experience, and functions (Nerenberg, 2002). The system, which applies to all paraprofessional workers regardless of the setting, would be a first step toward developing a uniform screening and quality assurance system. It would also be a first step in formalizing a "career ladder" for workers that could lead to fairer pay and heightened job satisfaction, which, in turn, would attract more individuals to the field.

As the result of an amendment to the Violent Crime and Law Enforcement Act of 1994, the U.S. attorney general developed guidelines to help states adopt safeguards to protect children, the elderly, or individuals with disabilities from abusive caregivers (U.S. Department of Justice, 1998). The guidelines emphasize that such factors as the vulnerability of the groups being served, the amount of time caregivers spend alone with their clients, whether they are monitored or supervised, and clients' ability to communicate should determine the amount of information that is collected prior to hiring. The guidelines recommend that caregivers' educational records; motor vehicle records; local, state, or FBI criminal records; and sex offender registries should always be checked. Additional information that should be obtained for caregivers who work with extremely vulnerable populations include psychological testing, alcohol or drug testing, and psychiatric history checks (U.S. Department of Justice, 1998). The report further recommends that professionals and advocates work with criminologists and researchers to develop screening measures for specific vulnerable populations. To date, this has not been done for elders. The need for research to guide hiring decisions is described in the next section.

RESEARCH CHALLENGES AND NEEDS

Research on elder abuse and neglect is critical to practice. To intervene effectively, those working with victims and perpetrator need information to help them understand the causes of abuse, its effects, and how they can help. Program developers and policy makers need compelling evidence on which to estimate the demand for services, the costs of services, and their anticipated impact. Perhaps the most pressing need is for studies that prove the effectiveness of services and interventions (Wolf, 1999a). This need has become particularly acute as governmental agencies and private funding sources become increasingly reluctant to support services whose effectiveness has not been demonstrated. The now ubiquitous term "evidence-based practice" refers to practices that have outcomes that are predictable, based on research, and that are known to be effective and beneficial.

The research on elder abuse has progressed slowly as a result of persistent problems that range from theoretical controversies to logistical glitches. The barriers researchers face in exploring outcomes are described in the next section. This is followed by a description of specific research needs.

Evaluating the Impact of Services

The need for research to establish what services, interventions, and therapeutic modalities work, for whom, and under what circumstances has been frequently voiced (Spencer, 1995; Stein, 1991; Tomita, 2006). Specifically, advocates and service providers have called for studies to explore the impact of APS, support groups, counseling, legal assistance, restitution recovery, daily money management, criminal prosecution, diversion programs, alternative dispute resolution, family conferencing, multidisciplinary teams, and batterer treatment programs. Also needed are studies to explore the impact of services on groups with special needs. This includes members of diverse cultural communities, and victims and abusers with mild, moderate, and severe dementias.

Evaluating services and interventions can be remarkably complex. Among the many obstacles that researchers face are difficulties defining success, translating practice goals into measurable outcomes, ethical concerns, and reticence by certain groups to participate in research.

Researchers need yardsticks with which to measure programs' successes. However, determining what those yardsticks should be is not always apparent. Clearly, stopping abuse or reducing its frequency and severity is a measure of success. But researchers recognize that victims may view the value of interventions and services differently (Spencer, 1995; Wolf &

Pillemer, 1989). Whereas removing an elderly victim from an abusive situation may stop the abuse, it may not be considered a successful intervention to a victim who does not want to move (Kozak, 1994).

Subjective perceptions of success are not dependable either. Many program evaluations solicit subjective feedback from clients about their level of satisfaction with services, asking if they believe they are better off as a result of the services and whether the benefits are worth the costs in terms of money, time, and the inconveniences they faced to participate. Other studies ask professionals to indicate changes they have noted in clients' behaviors or general well-being. Although these subjective measures of success provide valuable feedback to program personnel, they do not stand up to scientific scrutiny. Clients and service providers may express high levels of satisfaction with services that do not result in observable changes in clients' level of risk or well-being. Conversely, clients and professionals may fail to recognize, understand, or be able to articulate a program's impact.

On the other hand, researchers face formidable problems in conducting scientific evaluations. Determining conclusively that services or interventions work requires that victims be randomly assigned to receive them or not receive them. Those who do not receive them become "controls" and are studied for comparison purposes. The ethical acceptability of withholding potentially beneficial treatment from victims is among the obstacles researchers face in getting approval for studies from human subjects committees or institutional review boards at universities or research institutes (Paveza, 2002). Another ethical consideration that is likely to arise in elder abuse research is how to assess elderly subjects' capacity to agree to participate in studies.

A major gap in our understanding of services and interventions is their effectiveness for members of specific populations. One obstacle to conducting research on cultural variations is finding members of certain cultural communities who are willing to participate in research studies. For some, their reticence stems from distrust that is rooted in historical experiences. Also lacking are studies that explore the benefits of services and interventions for elders with cognitive impairments. It is obvious that new approaches and incentives are needed to achieve a clearer understanding of variations among diverse groups with respect to service utilization, the impact of services, patterns of help-seeking, and obstacles.

Developing practice-focused research requires give and take between researchers and service providers. To date, there have been few opportunities for researchers and service providers to engage in in-depth, focused exchange to explore unmet needs. Forums that attempted to promote this type of exchange have tended to be brief and limited in scope (Wolf, 1999). As a result, they yield plans and agendas that describe research needs in very broad strokes. What is needed are focused discussions aimed at generating hypotheses, sharing observations, identifying potential sources of data and subjects, and exploring ways to overcome barriers.

Assessing the Impact of Abuse Definitions on Practice

As stated earlier, practitioners need to understand how various definitions impact practice. For example, in deciding whether or not to use "functional criteria" to define eligibility for services (e.g., victims must be "vulnerable" or "dependent" as a result of cognitive, physical, and communication deficits), providers need to know how doing so will affect the size of their caseloads and their clients' service needs. Using functional criteria to determine eligibility for services further requires that agencies screen potential clients for deficits. The costs of screening must then be weighed against the costs of providing "universal coverage" to all victims over a certain age in making comparisons.

To a great extent, the information that advocates, program developers, and policy makers need to make informed decisions about definitions can be drawn from states' and agencies' experiences. State and agency surveys could, for example, shed light on:

- What states and agencies use functional requirements and why?
- How are the terms *dependent* and *vulnerable* defined, and what criteria and instruments are used to measure them?
- What are the costs associated with screening for dependency and vulnerability?
- How do the needs of dependent or vulnerable victims differ from other elderly victims?
- What are the costs of serving the two groups (i.e., elders with and without impairments)?

The Economic Costs of Elder Abuse

Few studies have attempted to analyze the costs associated with abuse and its treatment. This information is extremely important for advocates to have so that they can demonstrate and compare the costs and consequences of society's failure to address the problem with the costs and benefits of prevention. Major costs associated with abuse include the treatment of injuries, providing public benefits to those who become indigent as a result of abuse, and providing skilled nursing home care to elders who are no longer able to manage independently in the community as a result of abuse. Other primary costs associated with prevention and treatment include outreach; investigations; prosecuting offenders; and health, social, legal, and support services.

Cost analyses can also demonstrate the benefits of various approaches. For example, it can be demonstrated relatively easily that the prevention or early detection of pressure ulcers, a common outcome of neglect, can eliminate the need for weeks or months of intensive and expensive care.

Shedding Light on "Help-Seeking"

Although victims' tendency to refuse services and the barriers they face in seeking help have been common themes in the elder abuse literature, little is actually known about why elders refuse help, the barriers they face, their patterns of "help-seeking," what factors make them change their minds, and how service providers can encourage them to accept help. Specific areas that warrant exploration include the following:

- What factors determine if and when victims seek help? For example, do increases in the level of danger or decreases in their health status affect the likelihood that they will ask for help?
- Are elderly victims likely to seek out help multiple times before taking definitive steps to end their victimization? If so, how many times are they likely to do so, and does the response they receive from service providers affect subsequent decisions about seeking and accepting help?

Predicting Helpers' Risk of Abusing

As communities grapple with how to keep dangerous workers out of the long-term care workforce, they need guidance on which to base their decisions about hiring policies. Earlier in this chapter, it was noted that a 1998 report by the U.S. attorney general called for professionals and advocates to work with criminologists and researchers to develop screening measures for specific vulnerable populations, taking into account such factors as the setting in which care is provided, the level of monitoring, and clients' ability to communicate. A recent study by the Office of the Assistant Secretary for Planning and Evaluation (DHHS) that explored the relationship between past criminal background and subsequent abuse by nursing home employees also called for studies to guide hiring decisions (U.S. Department of Health and Human Services, 2006). In particular, research is needed about recidivism rates and what mitigating circumstances should be considered in hiring, such as employees' age at the time they committed crimes or the length of time since the crimes occurred.

Information that states and agencies need to inform hiring decisions and policy includes the following:

- What past criminal conduct is predictive of future abuse to seniors?
- What mitigating factors, such as the type of crime, the length of time since the criminal conduct occurred, and the perpetrators' participation in treatment or recovery programs, should be considered?

PROFESSIONAL TRAINING NEEDS

As the field of elder abuse prevention evolves, it has created a need for increasingly sophisticated training for an ever-growing pool of professionals and paraprofessionals.

Ensuring that professionals who are likely to encounter abuse have the information and training they need to recognize abuse and respond appropriately is complicated by the fact that new research findings and developments are emerging on an almost daily basis. Trainers with expertise in certain aspects of elder abuse and its prevention are in short supply. As the circle of mandated reporters, "sentinels," and "gatekeepers" widens, new groups need training. The abuse cases that service providers are encountering are becoming increasingly more diverse and complex. The turnover rates at many agencies and within certain professional groups are also high, creating a need for frequent, ongoing updates. In addition, competing demands on professionals' time and attention limits the amount of time they can devote to training. Because professionals from diverse disciplines may discover various forms of abuse in a variety of settings, the training they receive needs to reflect the situations they are likely to encounter.

Training needs assessments and practice experience have identified some unmet needs that are common to multiple groups and others that are specific to certain groups or settings. Examples of critical training needs for multiple groups include the following:

- Empowering victims to overcome obstacles to help
- Understanding clients' mental health needs
- The causes, treatment, prognosis, and symptoms of dementia, and the role of dementia in elder abuse
- Assessing clients' decision-making capacity for specific decisions

- Enhancing the decision-making capacity of elders with diminished capacity
- Assessing and "undoing" undue influence
- Principles and techniques associated with surrogate decision making
- How to serve as expert witnesses in criminal and civil abuse cases
- Financial abuse, including the following:
  - The dynamics between victims and perpetrators
  - How financial abuse relates to other forms of elder abuse
  - Strategies for investigating complex financial abuse such as abuse involving securities and annuities, living wills, and powers of attorney
  - The role of federal agencies in investigations, including the IRS, the Social Security Administration, the FBI, the U.S. Postal Service, the Secret Service, and U.S. attorneys
  - How financial predators operate, "red flags" that signal that elders have been targeted or are "chronic" victims, and whom to report to
- Legal, ethical, and practice issues associated with self-neglect

Examples of discipline-specific or cross-disciplinary training needs include the following:

- Judges can benefit from training to help them do the following:
  - Understand the importance of restitution for elderly victims
  - Evaluate "caregiver stress defenses"
  - Understand dementia, including its progression and how to determine when people are no longer culpable for their actions
  - Craft protective orders and guardianships that offer maximum protection and accountability
- Those working with caregivers need training to help them do the following:
  - Assess high-risk situations such as poor past relationships, previous histories of family violence, and caregivers' fears about becoming violent
  - Promote caregiver safety through safety checks and safety planning (including preventing people with dementias from accessing weapons)
- Medical professionals need training to help them do the following:
  - Distinguish inflicted injuries and abuse-related conditions from those that are the result of accidents or age-related causes

- Preserve medical forensic evidence and, in the case of emergency medical technicians and paramedics, crime scenes
- Recognize subtle behavioral indicators
- Local and federal victim/witness assistance advocates need the following:
  - Information about the elderly, their service needs, and available resources
  - Information on how to work with crime victims who have dementias

CHALLENGES TO COORDINATION AND COLLABORATION

Responding to abuse reports is a shared responsibility. This is true regardless of whether the abuse is criminal or not, and whether it occurs in long-term facilities or domestic settings. Those that share responsibility for investigating abuse reports need to coordinate their efforts so that they respond in a timely manner, evidence is preserved, and clients are not required to repeat their stories multiple times, causing unnecessary distress or trauma. When agencies that provide prevention services work together, it results in a more holistic and comprehensive response. When agencies collaborate on joint advocacy, outreach, and planning initiatives, it optimizes their resources and extends their influence.

Coordination and collaboration may be disrupted or impeded by many factors, including lack of clarity with respect to roles and responsibilities, competition for scarce resources, and tensions based on differences in perspective or ideology. Commonly cited conflicts with respect to roles and responsibilities include the following:

- Under federal law, LTC ombudsmen are mandated to serve as advocates for residents in long-term care facilities. Under their federal mandate, they cannot report abuse to APS or law enforcement unless they have residents' consent to do so (unless residents are incapable of giving consent). In some states, this federal prohibition conflicts with state laws that require LTC ombudsmen to report. The prohibition has also led to tensions between LTC ombudsmen, APS, and law enforcement.
- A few states mandate LTC ombudsmen to receive and investigate reports of abuse in facilities. This is in addition to their federal mandate to serve as advocates. Workers assigned to serve as both advocates and neutral fact finders may find these roles to be incompatible. In addition, this dual role may lead to the following conflicts:

- Lack of clarity with respect to what agency (LTC ombudsmen or APS) has responsibility for responding to abuse in the various types of long-term care facilities, including assisted living and intermediate care facilities. In some jurisdictions, the agencies' responsibilities overlap.
- When victims move between long-term care facilities and home (e.g., after acute hospitalizations), it may be unclear what agency has jurisdiction.

- Lack of clarity with respect to law enforcement jurisdiction. As more and more state and federal law enforcement agencies become involved in investigating and responding to elder abuse, determining what agency has jurisdiction has become increasingly difficult. For example, agencies with responsibility for investigating abuse in nursing homes include local law enforcement, Medicaid fraud control units, state regulatory and licensing agencies, the Centers for Medicare and Medicaid Services, the FBI, the U.S. Department of Justice, and the Office of the Inspector General. And agencies with responsibility for investigating fraud and identity theft may include the FBI, the Federal Trade Commission, the Social Security Administration, the Secret Service, and others.

Ideological differences or biases with respect to how cases should be handled can also lead to conflict. For example, advocates for victims or abusers are charged with representing or defending the interests of individual clients. These advocates may, therefore, find themselves in conflict with other professionals who work with multiple parties or whole families.

Barriers to information sharing can also impede coordination. Some professionals are unwilling to share information about clients because they believe it conflicts with professional ethics. Doctors, lawyers, bankers, and clergy, in particular, have argued that the mandatory duty to report abuse conflicts with their legal or ethical duties to maintain patient or client confidentiality.

Another frequently cited obstacle to information sharing is the federal Health Insurance Portability and Accountability Act (HIPAA) of 1996. The act was created to make it easier for employees with preexisting conditions to join employee-sponsored group health plans. In 2001, guidelines were published to clarify HIPAA's provisions for protecting patients' medical privacy. The guidelines set boundaries on how health records can be used and whom they can be released to. The new guidelines raised widespread concerns among many health care providers as to whether they could consult with other providers about patients' conditions without written authorization. Although the U.S. Department of Health Services stated that, "Consulting with another health care provider about a patient is within the HIPAA Privacy Rule's definition of 'treatment' and, therefore, is permissible," some health care providers (and other covered entities) have remained reticent to share information.

ETHICAL CHALLENGES

As the field of elder abuse prevention has evolved, it has, at times, led to a questioning of basic principles and values. Heightened scrutiny by the media and the sharp criticism it has sometimes engendered suggest that public perceptions about abuse and what should be done about it are not in sync with the perceptions and values of professionals with respect to client autonomy. When APS or others fail to intervene because capable victims have refused their help, the media, the public, and policy makers have at times been outraged. If the failure to intervene results in hardship, suffering, physical decline, losses, or tragedy, the criticism may be particularly harsh. The increasing frequency with which these events are occurring and the virulence of public disapproval suggests that the public in general has a lower tolerance for risk than the elders involved and those who serve them. As described in Chapter 4, some have suggested that the doctrines of self-determination and autonomy further need to be reassessed in light of an increasingly multicultural society in which not all cultural groups share the same values.

These apparent conflicts warrant further consideration. As we attempt to develop uniform and universal approaches to preventing abuse, it will become increasingly critical to build consensus.

CONCLUSION

The challenges described in this chapter are formidable. Meeting them requires that we take stock of where we have come from and develop a plan for the future. Specifically, we need to evaluate those services, models, and interventions that have already been put into place to determine which ones warrant expansion and replication. As new knowledge about services and victims' needs emerges, we need to interpret its implications and applications for public policy and service delivery. This new knowledge further needs to be integrated into practice at all levels so that victims, abusers, and family members receive state-of-the art services and interventions wherever they are and regardless of their circumstances. We also need to continue to explore and respond to services gaps and impediments to access. And finally, as the field matures, we also need to reconsider the basic guiding principles we have operated under to determine if they still apply and serve us well. The next and final chapter offers some suggestions for addressing these issues.

NOTE

1.For more on the Money Management Assistance Program, see http://www.hunter.cuny.edu/news/aging.shtml.

CHAPTER TEN

Moving Forward

INTRODUCTION

In the preface to this book, I quoted a colleague who doggedly urged our San Francisco network to devise a "master plan" to guide us. This chapter echoes and extends his appeal to the broader elder abuse prevention network. It further suggests some potential starting points. The chapter is part conceptual framework, part blueprint, and part "to do" list. It begins by proposing a set of overarching principles to guide service development and then suggests an approach, case management, which I believe offers the flexibility and tools that we need to serve clients effectively. And finally, I have proposed specific measures and steps to address some of the challenges and needs identified in the previous chapter.

GUIDING PRINCIPLES

In a field as complex and multifaceted as ours—and one that is as mired in slippery slopes, apparent contradictions, and clashing paradigms—there are no clear paths to follow in designing a response system. The best that we can hope for are principles to guide us. The principles I am suggesting are simple; they may even seem simplistic. Yet I believe that they can serve as guideposts to lead us forward and steer us back when we falter, diverge, or stray off course.

A comprehensive elder abuse service response system needs to do the following:

1. Take a holistic approach
2. Provide a continuum of service options

3. Address cultural differences
4. Employ a public health perspective and approach
5. Address victims' long-term, as well as emergency, service needs

1. A Holistic Response

The complexity of elder abuse has been widely acknowledged. In fact, the panel of experts, described in Chapter 2, that was convened by the National Academy of Sciences in 2002 to review and evaluate elder abuse research proposed an "ecological model" to accommodate the multiplicity of factors and theories associated with elder abuse (National Research Council, 2003). The ecological model has previously been applied to other forms of family violence and holds that violence results from a combination of individual, interpersonal, and societal factors (Schiamberg & Gans, 1999). It further acknowledges the interplay of these factors and how they contribute to risk.

Proposing this model was a somewhat radical step for the National Academy group. It was in sharp contrast to the numerous previous attempts by researchers, theorists, and service providers to find a single or primary cause or syndrome to explain elder abuse. Discussions about whether elder abuse is crime, a form of domestic violence, a public health problem, the result of ageism, a caregiver issue, or a social justice issue have often taken a decidedly competitive tone.

The ecological model acknowledges the multiple and complex factors that cause and trigger abuse, as well as the myriad physical, psychological, social, spiritual, and economic repercussions of these factors on the parties involved. Recognizing the complexity and interrelationships among these factors is an important first step. What's needed next is to acknowledge that solutions too must be interrelated; we need a holistic approach to prevention. This is not to suggest that we have not recognized that elder abuse calls for multiple interventions and services. Myriad solutions have been proposed, many of which are described in earlier chapters. But these services and interventions have typically been viewed as discrete and unrelated.

Holistic solutions to problems address their multiple causes and manifestations, and the interrelationships among the parties involved. A holistic response to elder abuse therefore is one that addresses the individual, interpersonal, and societal factors that give rise to abuse, as well as the physical, psychological, social, spiritual, and economic needs of victims, their families, and abusers. The needs of other vulnerable seniors and communities also need to be considered. A holistic response further requires that we look beyond formal support services and build upon the strengths, resources, and influence of victims' families, extended families, faith communities, and affinity groups.

And finally, a holistic approach to elder abuse must address the problem from a *macro*, as well as a *micro*, perspective. Whereas micro solutions focus on the problems and needs of individuals, macro solutions focus on the problems and needs of whole groups and institutions. Macro solutions also acknowledge and address the macro forces that contribute to problems, including economic factors and social injustices. Although our field has been shaped by such macro forces as the movement to serve increasingly frail elders in the community (as opposed to institutions), we have not paid much attention to how this development and others affect vulnerability or how to respond on a system level (e.g., how do we ensure that consumer choice programs offer adequate choices, protections, and recourse for vulnerable elderly consumers?). And although it has been frequently observed that elder abuse is found among members of all cultural, ethnic, gender, and economic groups, we have failed to seriously consider how such factors as discrimination, economic disadvantage, and social upheaval contribute to abuse, service needs, and access to services. Clearly, interventions with members of politically and economically disenfranchised groups have to focus on helping clients overcome economic and social barriers and exercise their rights. Collective advocacy is also needed to promote equal access to justice and resources.

Developing a holistic response will require changes in how agencies operate. For example, agencies may need to change policies to allow them to address the needs of multiple family members, share information, and work with clients' informal support networks. A holistic response will require us to extend our concept of perpetrator accountability beyond punishment and to create more opportunities for perpetrators to change their behavior, learn new skills, and make amends to their victims and communities though education, treatment, restitution, and community service. Agencies may further need to allow personnel to become involved in advocacy initiatives.

2. A Continuum of Service Options

As we begin to think holistically, we need to consider how services and interventions fit together in the big picture. For example, social, health, legal, and protective services vary in terms of the constraints they place on clients' autonomy and freedom. There is often a trade-off between safety and freedom; services that offer the greatest protection are likely to restrict clients' freedom, whereas services that maximize autonomy often involve significant risks. Therefore, interventions with victims may be viewed as falling along a continuum with respect to the restrictions they impose. The same is true for interventions and services for abusers. Programs that provide opportunities for abusers to stop abusing voluntarily fall on one end of a continuum, whereas forced separation from society through incarceration or confinement is on the other end.

Table 10.1 illustrates how services and interventions that may be needed to achieve various goals can be organized from least to most restrictive. (The list serves as an example. It is not exhaustive and the ranking of interventions with respect to restrictiveness may be subject to debate.)

Services can be organized in other ways or using other schemas. For example, an alternative continuum could reflect clients' abilities, with services for able-bodied seniors at one end and services for elders who are severely incapacitated at the other end. Similarly, services may be organized to reflect the severity of the abuse, with services that reduce risk on one end and emergency interventions on the other. The point is that services are interrelated and connected by unifying or overarching themes or goals. These themes and goals must be understood and accepted by the broader elder abuse prevention network.

3. Addressing Cultural Differences

In the past, there has been a tendency to address cultural differences by simply improving access to mainstream programs for members of underserved groups. In essence, this approach supposes that mainstream practices are appropriate for everyone.

This one-directional approach not only fails to acknowledge the important role that culture plays in dictating service needs, it also fails to acknowledge the insights and contributions that culturally specific programs have made to our field and their potential for replication or adaptation by mainstream programs. The following principles, approaches, and themes that have been identified by experts on cultural issues in elder abuse warrant further consideration.

- In developing services and interventions, agencies need to acknowledge and address cultural differences that may contribute to or mitigate risk. Factors to consider include the following:
  - Attitudes about aging and the role of elders in their families and communities
  - The roles and responsibilities of family members including the duty to provide care and financial support to elders
  - Experiences with racism, immigration, acculturation, disruption of family life, and other stresses
- Programs should reinforce cultural strengths and values. Specifically, programs and interventions should do the following:
  - Reinforce elders' roles in their families and communities
  - Promote intergenerational respect and empathy
  - Enlist the support of faith-based institutions
  - Build upon family strengths and relationships

Table 10.1 Intervention Options from Least to Most Restrictive

Goals	Services and Interventions (from least to most restrictive)
To reduce risk by enhancing frail elders' independence and ensuring that their daily needs are met	• Support services • Case management • Supervised or supportive housing, including senior residences and assisted living • Guardianship of person
To reduce the risk of financial abuse	• Education and information about finances, elder financial abuse, scams, etc. • Assistance executing advance directives including powers of attorney and trusts • Informal help with daily money management • Representative payeeship • Guardianship of estate
To ensure victim safety	• Monitor high-risk living arrangements (e.g., elders living with substance abusers) • Help victims plan for their own safety and consider options • Help victims take steps to ensure their safety; options include help finding shelter, legal assistance with restraining orders or evictions, terminating the employment of abusive live-in caregivers. • Remove perpetrators from victims' homes against victims' wishes through termination by third-party employers, court order, etc. • Involuntary, temporary removal of severely incapacitated victims into safe settings (e.g., through temporary guardianship or protective custody) to assess their health, mental health, or protective service needs • Involuntary, permanent removal of severely incapacitated victims from their homes into safe settings such as nursing homes when other options have been exhausted

To enhance the autonomy of elders with diminished decision-making capacity	• Enhance clients' decision-making capacity by helping them improve their health status
	• Supportive decision making
	• Surrogate decision making (in order of preference)
	  • Advance directives (elder has indicated wishes or preferences prior to the onset of incapacity)
	  • Substituted judgment
	  • Best interest

Table 10.1 *(Continued)*

Goals	Services and Interventions (from least to most restrictive)
Holding perpetrators accountable	• Voluntary treatment, education, and opportunities to make amends, including treatment for domestic violence and substance abuse; caregiver education • Programs that create incentives for perpetrators to participate in treatment or make amends to victims • Programs that compel offenders to receive treatment and make amends, including court-ordered treatment or restitution, etc. • Civil penalties • Confinement in locked psychiatric facilities or incarceration

- Strengthen informal caregiving networks through financial support, education, and conflict resolution
- Programs should enlist the support of nonabusive family, friends, and the community to reduce victims' reliance on perpetrators.
- Nonadversarial, nonpunitive options, such as mediation and family conferencing, should be available to resolve family conflicts when appropriate.
- Programs are needed that address social and economic factors such as the role of poverty and discrimination in abuse.

Mainstream programs stand to benefit from exploring how these principles apply or can be adapted. Some programs have already done so. For example, a few mainstream programs have adopted restorative justice techniques, including mediation and talking circles (family conferencing). Others have devised outreach campaigns that instill or reinforce respect for elders, acknowledge the contributions that elders make to their communities, and promote intergenerational understanding and exchange (see Chapter 8 for examples).

4. A Public Health Perspective

Addressing elder abuse as a public health problem offers new opportunities and tools. The public health field's emphasis on prevention provides an important counterbalance to our field's current emphasis on remedial legal and therapeutic interventions. Surveillance and epidemiological studies can help us achieve a clearer understanding of risk factors associated with abuse, which can help us identify high-risk groups to target for outreach and screening. It can also guide us in developing services to reduce the likelihood that abuse will occur in the first place or to catch it in the early stages when interventions can reduce pain, suffering, loss, decline, and dependency.

The public health approach offers intriguing possibilities for changing public attitudes and behaviors. Using social marketing and public health education techniques, public health campaigns can potentially shape attitudes about what is appropriate and inappropriate conduct by caregivers. They can influence attitudes about family members' duties to each other and the role of neighbors in looking out for vulnerable elders. Campaigns can further educate elders and families about techniques to reduce risk.

Public awareness campaigns that focus on promoting positive behavior (as opposed to campaigns that focus on generating reports to APS, police, or abuse hotlines) may meet with skepticism or resistance by professionals. This was the case when the Pennsylvania Department of Aging sought feedback prior to developing its "Elderly Pennsylvanians Deserve Honor and Respect" campaign. As described in Chapter 8, the department found that professionals preferred a hard-hitting campaign that encouraged reporting, whereas seniors favored the honor and respect approach. The seniors prevailed.

This reticence by professionals may suggest an underlying belief that efforts to promote positive behavior are too "soft" or vague to yield results. Yet, in fact, preventative approaches have had a powerful impact when applied to such serious public health problems as lung cancer, automobile accidents, and family violence. Public health education campaigns were largely responsible for dramatic changes in the public's attitudes and behaviors with respect to smoking, driving under the influence, and family violence.

Changing the public's attitudes will require us to consider such fundamental questions as what family members' role should be in caring for elders and what the public's role should be in identifying and responding to abuse and advocating for enlightened public policy. Specific questions that warrant consideration include the following:

- What attitudes does the public currently have about the elderly and abuse?
- Are there attitudes or public perceptions that need to change for elders to be safer and more secure? For example, do we need to clarify or establish what responsibility children have toward their elderly parents or educate the public about what is acceptable and unacceptable behavior?
- How do we translate what we have learned about help seeking to encourage victims to come forward, give them hope, gain their trust, and overcome their fears?

- What should we be telling witnesses about their roles and their responsibilities?
- What public policies do we want the public to advocate for?

5. Long-Term Services

Abuse prevention programs have traditionally focused on short-term interventions. APS, in particular, is viewed as a short-term intervention and many APS programs cap the number of visits workers can make or the period of time they can keep cases open. But as we achieve a clearer understanding of the help-seeking process and effective ways to treat abuse, it has become increasingly apparent that longer-term interventions are needed. We have come to understand, for example, that encouraging frightened, demoralized, ambivalent, or disenfranchised victims to take the steps needed to stop abuse may take weeks, months, or even years. It may require helping them work though denial, explore their options, resolve interpersonal conflicts, and reduce their risk of future abuse. Even after interventions have been completed, it may take time for victims to stabilize their situations, adapt to change, learn new behaviors, recover their losses, and heal from physical or emotional injuries. During this process, they are likely to need sustained contact and support. Long-term involvement with abusers may also be required to reinforce treatment and rehabilitation, hold them accountable for restitution or making amends, and prevent recurrences.

AN APPROACH: CASE MANAGEMENT

In some situations, abuse can be stopped through single remedial actions or through emergency and short-term interventions. Firing an abusive paid caregiver, for example, may be all that is needed to stop exploitation. But many elder abuse cases call for multiple interventions and sustained contact between clients and service providers. Victims, their families, and their abusers may require multiple services and interventions, and their needs may change over time. Their functional abilities, which dictate what services they need, may also fluctuate over time and, therefore, need to be continually reassessed. In these circumstances, case management offers a promising intervention option.

Case management, which is described in Chapter 5, was designed for people with disabilities who have multiple and changing needs. Its goal is to help clients achieve and maintain the highest level of independence possible. Case managers use functional and cognitive assessment tools to carefully monitor clients' ability to perform daily tasks, observe trends over time, and identify new service needs. Working with their clients and colleagues from other disciplines, case managers develop customized service plans and arrange for services. They perform routine follow-up assessments to monitor clients' progress and identify new needs or problems.

This approach can readily be applied to elder abuse and is compatible with the principles described above. For example, the model is holistic in that it addresses clients' multiple and interrelated needs, which may include the need for health and mental health care, legal aid, financial assistance, new housing, and support services. The focus of case management is on maximizing clients' independence and autonomy. This is accomplished by closely monitoring clients' abilities, matching services to needs, detecting problems during their early or incipient stages, and allowing for preventative measures or early treatment.

Adapting the case management model to elder abuse would require certain modifications. We would need to establish a new type of case manager, an "elder protection case manager." Elder protection case managers would require the following:

- Training to help them develop skills in both case management and elder abuse prevention. Elder protection case managers will need to be familiar with the techniques used to achieve both case management and protective service goals. The primary goals for case management programs are to maintain independence and prevent institutionalization. Although these goals also apply to the field of elder abuse prevention, elder protection case managers would further need to understand the "psychology of victimization" so that they can help victims work through denial, shame, guilt, and hopelessness. They must also be able to help victims withstand pressure, intimidation, and undue influence from abusers. Elder protection case managers also need skills in safety planning, crisis counseling, and legal advocacy and must be familiar with such commonly used abuse prevention interventions as restraining orders, shelters, and protective custody.
- Familiarity with both the case management and elder abuse prevention networks. Traditional case managers are accustomed to working with professionals from a wide range of disciplines and agencies. These include providers of health and mental health care, daily money management programs, probate courts, programs for caregivers, public benefits advocates, providers of support services and housing, and many others. But to effectively meet the needs of elder abuse victims, elder protection case managers would need

to extend their networks still further to include police, prosecutors, probation and parole officers, defense attorneys, domestic violence and victim service advocates, and others.

- Flexibility to work with victims' families, including perpetrators, when it is in clients' best interest to do so. Services that they may need include instruction and support in caregiving and mental health services, including treatment for depression and substance abuse.

- New assessment tools. The assessment tools that are currently used by case management programs include the Activities of Daily Living (ADL) and Instrumental Activities of Daily Living (IADL) scales, cognitive assessment instruments, and others. These tools are appropriate for elder abuse victims, whose functional abilities are also of critical importance in developing interventions. However, in addition, elder protection case managers would need to assess clients' risk and other abuse-related factors such as trauma and susceptibility to undue influence. Assessment tools would, therefore, need to be adapted or created to explore all of these factors.

Elder protection case management programs could be developed and operated either by APS programs or by public or private case management programs. The advantages and drawbacks of each would need to be considered. APS programs already have the authority, recognition, referrals, and experience needed to work with victims of elder abuse. Providing elder protection case management would, therefore, be a natural extension of what they already do. It would, however, require a significant infusion of resources. Case management programs, on the other hand, have the training, expertise, policies and procedures, tools, and infrastructures required by the model. They too, would need an infusion of resources to permit them to serve abused elders effectively.

AN AGENDA

Chapter 9 described a wide range of specific challenges our field faces with respect to research, training, advocacy, coordination, and outreach. This section proposes some "next steps" for addressing them.

Promoting Research

Throughout this book, I have repeatedly emphasized the need for practice-focused research. Our ability to craft a realistic plan for the future demands that we understand the scope of elder abuse, its impact, who is at risk, clients' service needs, and the effectiveness of existing services. This information is critical to designing services, targeting outreach and services to those at greatest risk, anticipating the demand for services, and demonstrating the need for resources and policy. Studies to demonstrate the effectiveness of programs are particularly crucial in this age of "evidence-based practice," as providers of private and public funding demand hard evidence attesting to programs' impact.

To foster this type of research, we need more opportunities for researchers and service providers to come together to share ideas and plan collaborative ventures. Improved communication is also critical. Just as service providers in our field have had to become conversant in the jargon of multiple disciplines, we must also learn how to communicate effectively with researchers, and vice versa. Both groups need to learn each other's terminologies, goals, and "tools of the trade."

Improved communication will benefit both researchers and service providers. Researchers can benefit from the practice wisdom of service providers, who can help them understand the nuanced goals of practice and the techniques they use. Workers' insights, observations, and hunches can be invaluable in helping researchers formulate hypotheses, predict results, and suggest explanations for equivocal findings. Service providers can further suggest promising avenues for exploration and identify potential data sources. When service providers see themselves as partners with researchers, they will be more willing to provide access to clients and to share resources and information.

Service providers also stand to gain from improved communication with researchers. Researchers can help practitioners understand research findings and interpret their implications and applications for practice. For instance, service providers need information about the incidence, prevalence, and risk factors associated with abuse to anticipate the demand for services, define target populations, and understand clients' needs. But for many service providers, the widely divergent findings yielded by incidence and prevalence studies are confusing. Researchers can help us understand why different methodologies and definitions lead to different findings and the implications of these differences. For example, studies that draw from agency records shed light on clients that agencies are likely to serve, whereas the findings of household surveys, which also capture abuse that is not reported, can reveal the needs of victims who are not known to the protective service system.

Elder abuse researchers and service providers may also potentially benefit from exchange and collaboration with their counterparts in other fields. Exchange with researchers and service providers in the field of domestic violence, for example, can help us better understand the goals and impact of the numerous services and interventions we have appropriated from that field, which include support groups, restraining orders, safety planning, and shelters. Collaboration with domestic violence researchers and advocates can also familiarize our network with the instruments and methods used to evaluate these interventions and services.

Similarly, elder abuse researchers and practitioners have much to offer our counterparts in other fields. For example, the research on consumer choice suggests that elderly consumers are less likely to be abused by caregivers they hire on their own than by helpers who work for agencies (Matthias & Benjamin, 2003). Clearly this research has critical implications for our field as we attempt to accommodate increasingly frail elders in our communities with a shrinking pool of home-care workers. Elder abuse researchers and service providers can potentially help interpret the findings of studies like these in light of what we know about risk factors that predict abuse. Discussions between the two networks could further point the way toward promising new areas of exploration.

This exchange can be achieved through formal or informal forums, ranging from brainstorming sessions to academic symposia. Electronic technology—including Listservs, Web sites, blogs, and electronic bulletin boards—can also help researchers identify practitioners with expertise in their areas of interest, clients who are willing to participate in studies, and other researchers with similar or related interests. In addition, practice-focused journals are needed that report on both the findings of elder abuse research and research from the fields of domestic violence, criminology, and caregiving that are relevant to our field. These journals could provide opportunities for practitioners and researchers to share their observations, experiences, findings, and insights in a more in-depth way and on an ongoing basis.

The need for scientific studies to demonstrate the impact of elder abuse prevention services and to guide program developers in the replication of effective practices has also been frequently noted. A potentially promising model for promoting program evaluation and replication is the "Blueprints for Violence Prevention" project, which was initiated in 1996 by the Center for the Study and Prevention of Violence (CSPV) at the University of Colorado at Boulder. The project identifies violence prevention and intervention programs that meet a strict scientific standard of program effectiveness in reducing adolescent violent crime, aggression, delinquency, and substance abuse. Center personnel, in consultation with an advisory board that comprises experts in the field of violence prevention, review programs to determine whether they meet three criteria: (1) there is evidence, supported by scientific research, that the programs deter violence; (2) there is evidence that positive changes are sustained over time; and (3) the programs have been replicated. To qualify as "blueprints," programs must meet all three criteria. To qualify as "promising programs," they only have to meet the first criterion.

In addition to identifying promising models, the Blueprints for Violence Prevention project provides training and technical assistance to help communities set up new programs. Designers of the blueprint and model programs provide training and consultation to sites that are replicating their programs. CSPV monitors the replication process to identify and respond to problems the new programs face. CSPV further explores factors that predict the success of replications, such as the organizational capacity, funding stability, commitment, and resources of the agencies replicating the models.[1]

As agencies and organizations around the world develop new programs to prevent and treat elder abuse, models like the Blueprints for Violence Prevention program clearly should be explored.

Training

Seeing to it that victims and the vulnerable get the services they need requires that professionals who work with the elderly recognize abuse and high-risk situations and respond appropriately. Chapter 9 described some of the challenges our field faces in ensuring that professionals have the training they need to do so. It further identified some of our most pressing training needs.

These challenges and gaps call for new technologies and approaches. We need, for example, approaches that reflect the diverse settings in which professionals work and the different types of abuse they are likely to encounter. Training can also be enriched by drawing from the knowledge and expertise of those being trained. In addition, we need new technologies to extend the "reach" of the limited pool of experts in some aspects of elder abuse. These include experts in institutional abuse, capacity and undue influence assessment, sexual assault, self-neglect, abuse investigation, clinical approaches to treatment, financial abuse, and others.

To achieve these objectives, elder abuse training programs are increasingly applying adult learning techniques and computer technology. Adult learning theory is based on the assumption that adults have special needs and requirements as learners. To be of value to adults, learning has to be applicable to their lives. Applying the concept to professional training means that training has to reflect the settings in which professionals work. Adult learning theory further acknowledges that adults have accumulated a foundation of life experiences and knowledge from which they can draw. To capitalize on students' expertise, adult education programs employ techniques like interactive problem-solving exercises that permit students to work with colleagues from the same field or agency, or from other fields and agencies, to enrich the learning experience. Specifically, professional training in elder abuse may include opportunities for students to work in teams to review case studies, plan interventions, and learn how cases are assessed by other disciplines.

Computer technology, including interactive Web-based programs, is also increasingly being used to train professionals in the field of elder abuse. Distance learning permits learners to benefit from a limited pool of experts. Interactive computer training allows students to work at their own pace, customize training to meet their individual needs, and participate at their convenience. Some computer-based training programs provide immediate feedback to reinforce learning.

Improving the quality and accessibility of training will undoubtedly encourage more professionals to take part. However, additional incentives are still needed. Professionals are most likely to participate in training programs that are taught by professionals from their own fields or disciplines and that are conducted, sponsored, or endorsed by organizations they trust. Trusted sources of training include local, state, and national professional associations; political figures, including governors and attorneys general; universities; and training institutes. Professionals are also more likely to participate if they receive continuing education credit.

As described in Chapter 7, some states have mandated training for certain groups. In order for training to reach an even wider audience, advocates can appeal to professional and licensing organizations to make elder abuse training compulsory. National and state organizations that oversee the distribution of training funds, including Victims of Crime Act (VOCA) and Violence Against Women Act (VAWA) funds, can also be asked to prioritize training in elder abuse.

The following principles can serve to guide the development of training in elder abuse:

- Training should be both discipline specific and interdisciplinary. Discipline-specific training permits professionals from the same discipline to share insights, learn from each other's experiences, and identify resources. Trainers can tailor the content to focus on their audiences' specific informational needs and specific situations that trainees are likely to encounter. On the other hand, interdisciplinary training can help students better understand the approaches used by other disciplines and promote ongoing interdisciplinary exchange.
- Training should employ the principles and methods of adult learning to reflect the knowledge, experiences, and expertise of

trainees. Specific techniques include problem solving exercises and role-playing.

- Computer technology should be used to enhance training. This includes computer-enhanced training, which allows students to spend time in the classroom but also provides them with online interactive exercises that permit them to test their skills or knowledge. They can also interact with other students or instructors through "chat rooms" or bulletin boards. An alternative is "distance learning" in which most or all work is completed online.

Filling Service Gaps

As new service gaps are identified, advocates need to decide how to fill them in the most effective and cost-efficient way. In some instances, this may mean working with mainstream programs—such as shelters, support groups, counseling programs, legal service providers, and others—to extend coverage to elderly clients. Alternatively, service gaps can be filled by existing aging and adult protective service programs. In still other instances, new programs or services are needed. Each approach offers advantages and disadvantages and raises critical concerns, which are described below.

Adapting Mainstream Programs to Meet the Needs of Abused Elders

Adapting mainstream programs for elders may require improving access and making programmatic changes. The widespread interest in domestic violence prevention by our network, which began in the mid-1990s, prompted many communities to explore elderly victims' need for shelter, restraining orders, support groups, counseling, and other services. As a starting point, many advocates turned to mainstream domestic violence and victim assistance providers to see if they were currently serving elderly victims or if they were willing or able to do so. What they found was that few mainstream programs were serving elders or doing so adequately (AARP, 1994; Vinton, 1998). The reasons were varied. Domestic violence programs and shelters have traditionally been required by their sponsors to focus on younger women with children. Additionally, advocates who work in mainstream programs are not generally trained in working with the elderly. They are, therefore, unlikely to be aware of elders' specific needs or how services need to be adapted for the elderly population. For instance, legal aid programs that focus on younger clients may not be aware of the repercussions that divorce can have on victims' retirement income, housing, and health insurance. Despite these problems, many mainstream domestic violence programs began providing services such as shelter, support groups, and counseling to older women as described in Chapter 5. In some instances, these efforts have been successful, as the following example demonstrates:

> We had an elderly woman come to our shelter, and it was amazing. She was very disabled but really bonded with the younger women. They respected the courage it took for her to finally leave an abusive husband after many years. She was an inspiration to them. Meeting a woman in her 70s who'd been battered for decades was also a reality check for the younger residents who believed that their own abusers would eventually stop. (Advocate in a battered women's shelter)

Chapter 5 also cites a study by the Older Women's Network in Ontario, which suggests that older women are not as concerned as service providers are about the potential problems involved in serving young and old victims together (Older Women's Network, n.d.). The adaptation of mainstream domestic violence programs to serve elderly victims clearly warrants further discussion.

Mainstream offender treatment programs have also successfully integrated perpetrators of elder abuse into their programs (see Chapter 5 for an example). However, the facilitator of another men's treatment group recalls the problems his organization encountered in doing so:

> When we got a referral for a younger man who had abused his mother, the group didn't accept him. They felt their issues weren't the same. So we had him see an individual counselor. But the counselor eventually determined that he was not able to address the client's severe emotional problems either. (Counselor in a treatment program for men)

In considering whether to adapt mainstream programs to accommodate elderly clients, the following factors need to be considered:

- Are mainstream programs willing and able to serve elders? Are they prevented from doing so by law, regulation, or restrictions imposed by funding sources?
- What new skills and resources do their staff need? For example, what information do they need about the aging process, detecting and responding to common deficits, and the aging services network?
- Is there a "cutoff" point with respect to clients' physical and mental capacity, at which mainstream agencies can no longer serve elderly victims effectively?
- Are elderly victims comfortable interacting with younger victims? Are younger clients accepting of elderly ones?

Expanding Aging and Adult Protective Service Programs'
Capacity to Fill Gaps

In some communities, aging and APS programs have developed new services to help fill service gaps. For example, as described in Chapter 5, nursing homes and assisted living facilities in several communities provide emergency shelter to victims.

In determining whether aging and APS programs can or should be expanded to fill service gaps, the following factors need to be considered:

- Are there obstacles to doing so? Are APS and aging service programs prevented from providing services needed by victims by law, regulation, or funding sources? If so, can these obstacles be overcome (e.g., residential care facilities have been able to secure special waivers to accept clients on an emergency basis without the paperwork and medical clearance that is normally required).
- What additional new skills and resources do the staff of APS and aging service programs need to extend the scope of services they provide to elderly victims? For example, what information do they need about elder abuse, domestic violence, help seeking, safety planning, and crisis intervention?
- What additional measures do they need to take to ensure client safety?
- Is there a cutoff point at which traditional aging service programs cannot serve victims effectively (e.g., when victims' need for special security measures exceeds what they can realistically provide)?

Strategies to Fund Services to Fill Gaps

Regardless of what agencies fill service gaps, new resources will be needed. Sources of funding and strategies for meeting new needs are described below. The benefits and drawbacks of various approaches are also described.

- Government: Several state and local legislatures, executives, and departments have allocated funds for new services or to supplement existing services. The new funds may be allocated at the urging of senior advocacy organizations, state or local abuse prevention coalitions, or professional associations. New services may be funded through general funds or by special measures such as surtaxes, fees (e.g., on death certificates), or requests for contributions on state income taxes. The main benefit of public allocations is that they are often substantial and ongoing. In addition, public entities can dictate how services are to be provided, leading to greater consistency. On the other hand, the extensive regulations and restrictions that may also be imposed can limit a programs' flexibility. In addition, securing public funds typically requires new legislation, which is extremely time-consuming and labor-intensive.

- Model projects and start-up funds: States, federal agencies, and nongovernmental sources, including foundations and the United Way, have funded model projects and provided start-up funds to explore promising new services. For example, in the 1990s, the Administration on Aging provided funds to local, state, and federal organizations to develop services for older battered women. An advantage of such programs is that they typically allow for significant flexibility in designing services and modifying them as new needs or obstacles are encountered. Model projects must typically collect data to demonstrate their impact and disseminate their findings and products. Additionally, model projects and start-up funds are time-limited, and program administrators must, therefore, find ways to sustain programs.
- Extending eligibility to, or prioritizing, abused elders: Agencies may modify their eligibility criteria or priorities to include abused elders who would not otherwise qualify. For example, case management programs that target elders who are at risk for nursing home placement may broaden their eligibility criteria to include elders who are at risk for abuse, neglect, and self-neglect.
- Public-private partnerships: Nonprofit agencies are increasingly working with for-profit organizations to develop services. For example, in some communities, private attorneys and professional fiduciaries have agreed to take some elder abuse cases on a pro bono basis. As noted previously, private hospitals and residential care facilities have agreed to provide emergency shelter.

Advocacy

Elder abuse advocacy at the national level has focused on alerting federal legislators to the need for services, the costs and burdens to society of failing to prevent abuse, and the lack of parity between protective services for elders and other victims of family violence. Specifically, they have concentrated on increased funding for the Social Services Block Grant (SSBG) program.

The Elder Justice Act, which was originally introduced in 2002 and reintroduced in subsequent sessions, has also been a focal point for national advocacy. The current version boosts funding for the LTC Ombudsman Program, establishes an APS grant program and forensics centers, and creates a coordinating council of federal agencies to make policy recommendations and submit reports to Congress every two years. The legislation further requires the Departments of Labor and Health and Human Services to take a proactive role in funding initiatives aimed at improving training programs and working conditions for long-term care professionals as a strategy for increasing the number of workers.

As momentum for establishing a comprehensive and uniform national response builds, the need to be prepared with a clear vision and plans for implementing it is increasingly critical. Beyond advocating for a comprehensive elder abuse law, I believe we also need to explore how other federal programs and policy that impact the elderly can support our efforts and reduce the risk of abuse. I further believe that our efforts to promote positive change can be enhanced by building partnerships and alliances with other advocacy networks. I have offered a few suggestions for doing so.

Exploring the Potential Role of Federal Agencies and Programs

As described above, elder abuse advocacy at the federal level has focused on securing additional funds for APS, LTC ombudsmen, and elder abuse prevention efforts. Although these efforts are of the utmost importance, there are other promising avenues that have received less attention. Although limited in scope, the following steps can potentially have a significant impact.

- Encourage or require federally funded programs for elders and caregivers to screen for the risk of abuse and neglect and prioritize high-risk seniors and/or their families for services. Examples include programs funded under the National Family Caregiver Support Program and Medicaid funded case management programs.
- Require federal employees, including U.S. postal workers, U.S. attorneys, FBI and FTC personnel, and others to report suspected abuse under state reporting statutes (federal employees currently must report child abuse).
- Appeal to Health and Urban Development (HUD) officials to prioritize abused or vulnerable elders for subsidized housing when they have been left homeless as a result of abuse or when the lack of housing keeps victims in abusive relationships.
- Permit Medicare and Medicaid funds to be used for abuse-related health and mental health services including counseling, the treatment of abuse-related trauma, and short-term hospital stays for

frail victims who need emergency shelter when other shelters cannot meet their care needs.

Collaborating with Other Advocacy Networks

Advocates in the field of elder abuse prevention also have much to gain from collaborating with other networks and disciplines to achieve common advocacy goals. By developing partnerships in advocacy at the local, state, tribal, national, and international levels, we can consolidate resources, benefit from strength in numbers, and defuse conflict and competition. Examples of potential partners and promising areas of collaboration include the following:

- **Collaboration with advocates for family caregivers, persons with disabilities, and consumer choice is needed to do the following:**
  - Address the critical shortage of home-care workers and workers in long-term care facilities that exists in many communities. This may be accomplished by advocacy to raise workers' wages, improve working conditions, institute quality control measures, and develop effective approaches to recruitment.
  - Develop effective mechanisms for screening and monitoring workers, and responding to reports of abuse by workers. Specific areas of need include laws that provide for background checks, protocols for responding to reports, and registries of offenders.
- **Collaboration with mental health advocates is needed to do the following:**
  - Address the critical shortage of services for both elders and nonelderly adults with mental health problems, including mental illnesses, dementias, and substance abuse. Specific services that are needed include age-appropriate treatment programs, daily money management, housing, guardians, and guardian monitors. Also needed are age-appropriate services for families of persons with mental health problems.
  - Find appropriate and humane options to prevent abuse by violent persons with dementias and mental illnesses, including secured facilities.
  - Ensure that victims and perpetrators with mental health problems who become involved in the criminal justice system are treated fairly and humanely.
- **Collaboration with victims' rights advocates is needed to do the following:**
  - Advocate for federal and state legislation that benefits victims of crime. Specific examples include supporting the proposed

victims' rights amendment to the U.S. Constitution and restitution reform measures. Collaborative advocacy can also focus on increasing funding for Victims of Crime Act (VOCA) programs. This can be accomplished by urging the government to more aggressively enforce the collection of federal criminal fines, forfeited bail bonds, and court assessments owed by federally convicted criminal offenders, all of which are used to fund VOCA programs.

- Support initiatives to achieve greater parity for victims of financial crimes who have not traditionally received many of the same services as victims of violent crimes.
- Promote the development of age-appropriate victim services.
- **Collaboration with domestic violence advocates is needed to do the following:**
  - Increase funding for Violence Against Women Act (VAWA)
  - Address the impact of the *Crawford* decision (see Chapter 7) on prosecuting perpetrators of domestic violence and elder abuse
  - Ensure that domestic violence advocates and those working in the justice systems understand the special needs of elderly victims of domestic violence and the needs of their abusers; specific areas of concern include the treatment of elderly victims and perpetrators of intimate partner abuse with dementias

CONCLUSION

The field of elder abuse prevention is at a critical juncture. New opportunities for affecting significant change are arising at the local, state, national, and international levels. For the first time, we have the attention of lawmakers, the media, and the public. To take full advantage of these unprecedented opportunities, we need a plan for the future.

Our field has drawn from many traditions, movements, and ideologies. These sources have suggested myriad explanations for abuse and just as many solutions. They suggest far-ranging approaches to prevention: from changing how society views old age, to resolving interpersonal conflicts; from demanding equal access to services and justice for elders, to enhancing the penalties we impose on criminals who prey on the vulnerable. Drawing from these sources, we have improvised and experimented, which has resulted in a striking array of services, interventions, and policies.

This diversity, though, is both a blessing and a curse. Although it has enriched our field and provided an abundance of resources, insights, and opportunities, it has also made it difficult to achieve a common vision and goals. This, in turn, has impeded our ability to construct a coherent and comprehensive service response system. It has stymied advocacy, frustrated lawmakers and the public, and led to divisions within our own ranks.

As we enter a new stage in our development, we need to find common ground and a common vision. This does not mean looking for simple solutions. They do not exist. Neither is there a single approach, a single agency, or a single discipline equipped to do everything that is needed. There are no protocols or algorithms that fit all situations. The best that we can hope for are guiding principles we can agree upon and turn to for guidance and inspiration. The principles advanced in this chapter are offered as a starting point. They capitalize on our diversity and use it to our advantage.

But although principles can steer us forward and keep us on track, they do not supplant the need for open communication and dynamic exchange within our ranks and beyond. We need to continue to build and strengthen our network and forge new alliances at the local, state, national, and international levels. We also need to create new forums and more opportunities to deliberate, plan, air differences, engage in problem solving, and build consensus. This chapter has suggested just a few of the issues we need to address, who might be our best allies and partners, and opportunities for working together to affect change. The themes of collaboration, inclusiveness, and open exchange resound throughout this book; it is therefore appropriate that I end with them. It is only through the sharing of ideas, expertise, and resources—both among ourselves and with those in related disciplines—that we can hope to achieve security and justice for elders.

NOTE

1. For more on the "Blueprints" project, see http://www.colorado.edu/cspv/blueprints/.

References

AARP. (1994). *Survey of services for older battered women: Final report.* Washington D.C.: AARP.

AARP. (1996). *Telemarketing fraud and older Americans: An AARP survey.* Washington D.C.

AgeingNet. (2002). Summary of INSTRAW electronic discussion forum on gender aspects of violence and abuse of older persons. Retrieved December 9, 2006, from the WWW: http://www.un-instraw.org/en/research/ageing/docs/Instraw_Summary_complete_version.pdf

Aitkin, L., & Griffin, G. (1996). *Gender issues in elder abuse.* London: Sage.

Allison, E. J., Ellis, P. C., & Wilson, S. E. (1998). Elder abuse and neglect: The emergency medicine perspective. *European Journal of Emergency Medicine, 5*(3), 355–363.

American Association of Retired Persons. (1992). *Abused elders or older battered women?* Washington D.C.: AARP.

American Association of Retired Persons. (1996). National survey of daily money management programs: A survey by the American Association of Retired Persons. Washington D.C.: Author.

American Bar Association Commission on Law and Aging, American Psychological Association, & National College of Probate Judges. (2006). *Judicial determination of capacity of older adults in guardianship proceedings: A handbook for judges.* Retrieved June 19, 2007, from http://www.abanet.org/aging/docs/judges_book_5-24.pdf

American Medical Association. (1992). *Diagnostic and treatment guidelines on elder abuse and neglect.* Chicago: AMA.

American Prosecutors Research Institute. (2003). *Fifty-one experiments in combating elder abuse: A digest of state laws on elder abuse, neglect, and exploitation.* Alexandria: American Prosecutors Research Institute.

Anetzberger, G. J. (1987). *The etiology of elder abuse by adult offspring.* Springfield, IL: C.C. Thomas.

Anetzberger, G. J. (1997). Elderly adult survivors of family violence. Implications for clinical practice. *Violence against Women, 3*(5), 499–514.

Anetzberger, G. J. (2005). The reality of elder abuse. In G. J. Anetzberger (Ed.), *The clinical management of elder abuse* (pp. 1–25). New York: Haworth.

Anetzberger, G. J., Korbin, J. E., & Austin, C. A. (1994). Alcoholism and elder abuse. *Journal of Interpersonal Violence, 9*(2), 184–193.

Ascione, F. R., & Arkow, P. (Eds.). (1999). *Child abuse, domestic violence, and animal abuse: Linking the circles of compassion for prevention and intervention.* West Lafayette, IN: Purdue University Press.

Aziz, S. J. (2000). Los Angeles county fiduciary abuse specialist team: A model for collaboration. *Journal of Elder Abuse & Neglect, 12*(2), 79–83.

Aziz, S. J., Bolick, D. C., Kleinman, M. T., & Shadel, D. P. (2000). The National Telemarketing Victim Call Center: Combating telemarketing fraud in the U.S. *Journal of Elder Abuse & Neglect, 12*(2), 93–101.

Baldridge, D. (2002). *The needs of Indian elders: A hearing by the Senate Committee on Indian Affairs. Statement by the National Indian Council on Aging.* Retrieved August 29, 2007, from http://www.senate.gov/~scia/2002hrgs/071002hrg/baldridge.PDF

Beach, S. R., Schulz, R., Williamson, G. M., Miller, L. S., Weiner, M. F., & Lance, C. E. (2005). Risk factors for potentially harmful informal caregiver behavior. *Journal of the American Geriatrics Society, 52*(2), 255–261.

Benton, D. (1998). Risk factors for elder mistreatment among African-Americans. In The Archstone Foundation (Ed.), *Understanding and combating elder abuse in minority communities* (pp. 123–130). Long Beach: Archstone Foundation.

Bergeron, L. R. (1999). Decision-making and adult protective services workers: Identifying critical factors. *Journal of Elder Abuse & Neglect, 10*(3/4), 87–113.

Bergeron, L. R. (2001). An elder abuse case study: Caregiver stress or domestic violence? You decide. *Journal of Gerontological Social Work, 34*(4), 47–63.

Bergeron, L. R. (2002). Family preservation: An unidentified approach in elder abuse protection. *Families in Society: The Journal of Contemporary Human Services, 83*(5/6), 547–556.

Bergeron, L. R., & Gray, B. (2003). Ethical dilemmas of reporting suspected elder abuse. *Social Work, 48*(1), 96–105.

Benecke, M., Josephi, E., & Zweihoff, R. (2004). Neglect of the elderly: Forensic entomology cases and considerations. *Forensic Science International, 146 Suppl.,* S195–199.

Binational Working Group on Cross-Border Mass-Marketing Fraud. (2003). *Mass-marketing fraud: A report to the Attorney General of the United States and the Solicitor General of Canada.* Retrieved March 27, 2007, from http://www.usdoj.gov/opa/pr/2003/May/remmffinal.pdf

Blenkner, M., Bloom, M., Nielson, M., & Weber, R. D. (1974). *Final report: Protective services for older people, findings from the Benjamin Rose Institute study.* Cleveland, OH: The Benjamin Rose Institute.

Blunt, A. (1993). Financial exploitation of the incapacitated: Investigation and remedies. *Journal of Elder Abuse & Neglect, 5*(1), 19–32.

Bradshaw, D., & Spencer, C. (1999). The role of alcohol in elder abuse cases. In J. Pritchard (Ed.), *Elder abuse work: Best practice in England and Canada* (pp. 332–353). London: Jessica Kingsley.

Brandl, B., Dyer, C. B., Heisler, C. J., Otto, J. M., Stiegel, L. A., & Thomas, R. (2007). *Elder abuse detection and intervention*. New York: Springer.

Brandl, B., Hebert, M., Rozwadowski, J., & Spangler, D. (2003). Feeling safe, feeling strong: Support groups for older abused women. *Violence against Women, 9*(12), 1490–1503.

Breckman, R., & Adelman, R. (1988). *Strategies for helping victims of elder mistreatment*. Newbury Park: Sage Publications.

Brogdon, B. G. (1998). *Forensic Radiology*. Boca Raton, FL: CRC Press.

Brown, A. (1998). A service provider perspective of Native American elder abuse: A research report. In The Archstone Foundation (Ed.), *Understanding and combating elder abuse in minority communities* (pp. 97–112). Long Beach: Archstone Foundation.

Brownell, P., Berman, J., & Salamone, A. (1999). Mental health and criminal justice issues among perpetrators of elder abuse. *Journal of Elder Abuse & Neglect, 11*(4), 81–94.

Brownell, P., & Heiser, D. (2006). Psycho-educational support groups for older women victims of family mistreatment: A pilot study. *Journal of Gerontological Social Work, 46*(3/4).

Brownmiller, S. (1975). *Against our will: Men, women and rape*. New York: Simon and Shuster.

Brozowski, K., & Hall, D. (2004). Growing old in a risk society. *Journal of Elder Abuse & Neglect, 16*(3), 65–81.

Burgess, A. W., & Clements, P. T. (2006). Information processing of sexual abuse in elders. *Journal of Forensic Nursing, 2*(3), 113–120.

Burgess, A. W., Dowdell, E. B., & Prentky, R. A. (2000). Sexual abuse of nursing home residents. *Journal of Psychosocial Nursing & Mental Health Services, 38*(6), 10–18.

Cambridge, P., & Parkes, T. (2004). The case for case management in adult protection. *Journal of Adult Protection, 6*(2), 4–14.

Chang, J., & Moon, A. (1997). Korean American elderly's knowledge and perceptions of elder abuse: A qualitative analysis of cultural factors. *Journal of Multicultural Social Work, 6*(1/2), 139–154.

Cohen, D. (1998). Homicide-suicide in older persons. *American Journal of Psychiatry, 155*, 390–396.

Cohen, D. (2000). An update on homicide-suicide in older persons: 1995–2000. *Journal of Mental Health and Aging, 6*(3), 195–197.

Coker, D. (1999). Enhancing autonomy for battered women: Lessons from Navajo peacemaking. *UCLA Law Review, 47*(1), 1–111.

Coker, D. (2002). Transformative justice: Anti-subordination processes in cases of domestic violence. In H. Strang & J. Braithwaite (Eds.), *Restorative justice and family violence* (pp. 128–152). Melbourne: Cambridge University Press.

Coker, D. (2004). Race, poverty, and the crime centered response to domestic violence: A comment on Linda Mill's, insult to injury, rethinking our responses to intimate abuse. *Violence Against Women, 10*(11), 1331–1353.

Coleman, V. (1994). Lesbian battering: The relationship between personality and the perpetration of violence. *Violence and Victims, 9*(2), 139–152.

Collingridge, M., & Miller, S. (1997). Filial responsibility and the care of the aged. *Journal of Applied Philosophy, 14*(2), 119.

Collins, K. A., & Presnell, S. E. (2006). Elder homicide: A 20-year study. *American Journal of Forensic Medicine & Pathology, 27*(2), 183–187.

Compton, S. A., Flanagan, P., & Gregg, W. (1997). Elder abuse in people with dementia in Northern Ireland: Prevalence and predictors in cases referred to a psychiatry of old age service. *International Journal of Geriatric Psychiatry, 12*(6), 632–635.

Cooney, C., & Mortimer, A. (1995). Elder abuse and dementia: A pilot study. *International Journal of Social Psychiatry, 41*, 276–283.

Coyne, A. C., Reichman, W. E., & Berbig, L. J. (1993). The relationship between dementia and elder abuse. *American Journal of Psychiatry, 150*(4), 643–646.

Dahlberg, L. L., & Krug, E. G. (2002). Violence: A global public health problem. In E. Krug, L. L. Dahlberg, J. A. Mercy, A. B. Zwi, & R. Lozano (Eds.), *World Report on Violence and Health.* (pp. 1–56). Geneva, Switzerland: World Health Organization.

Daly, J., & Jogerst, G. (2001). Statute definitions of elder abuse. *Journal of Elder Abuse & Neglect, 13*(4), 39–57.

Daly, K., Curtis-Fawley, S., Bouhours, B., Weber, L., & Scholl, R. (2003). *Sexual offence cases finalised in court, by conference and by formal caution in South Australia for young offenders, 1995–2001.* Retrieved November 17, 2006, from http://www.griffith.edu.au/school/ccj/kdaly.html

Davis, R., & Medina-Ariza, J. (2001). *Results from an elder abuse prevention experiment in New York City.* Washington D.C.: U.S. Department of Justice, National Institute of Justice.

Dawson, J. D., & Langan, P. (1994). *Murder in families.* Washington, DC: Bureau of Justice Statistics, U.S. Department of Justice.

Dean Crisp, S. M. (2002). *Old age is not for cowards: Increased vulnerability to elder abuse through grief and other losses.* Retrieved August 29, 2007, from www.onpea.org/en/SideNavigation/Publications/ConferenceProceedings/conference04/25DeanCrisp.pdf

de Benedictis, T., Jaffe, J., & Segal, J. (2004). Elder abuse types, signs, symptoms, causes, and help. Retrieved June 6, 2006, from http://www.helpguide.org/mental/elder_abuse_physical_emotional_sexual_neglect.htm

Deem, D. L. (2000). Notes from the field: Observations in working with the forgotten victims of personal financial crimes. *Journal of Elder Abuse & Neglect, 12*(2), 33–48.

Deem, D., Nerenberg, L., & Titus, R. (2007). Victims of financial crime. In R. C. Davis, A. J. Lurigio, & S. Herman (Eds.), *Victims of crime* (3rd ed.) (pp. 125–145). Thousand Oaks, CA: Sage Publications.

Doolity, C., & Greenberg, M. (2003). *Adult protective services: Responding to financial exploitation of vulnerable adults.* Retrieved May 17, 2007, from http://www.governmentlaw.org/files/adult_protect_services.pdf

Drayton-Hargrove, S. (2000). Assessing abuse of disabled older adults: A family system approach. *Rehabilitation Nursing, 25*(4), 136–140.

Duke, J. (1991). A national study of self-neglecting adult protective services clients. In T. Tatara & M. Rittman (Eds.), *Findings of five elder abuse studies* (pp. 23–53). Washington D.C.: National Aging Resource Center on Elder Abuse.

Dundorf, K., & Brownell, P. (1995). When the victim is elderly. *The Family Advocate, 17*(3), 81–83.

Dyer, C. B., Connolly, M. T., & McFeeley, P. (2003). The clinical and medical forensics of elder abuse and neglect. In R. J. Bonnie & R. B. Wallace (Eds.), *Elder mistreatment: Abuse, neglect, and exploitation in an aging America* (pp. 339–381). Washington, DC: National Academies Press.

Dyer, C. B., Pavlik, V. N., Murphy, K. P., & Hyman, D. J. (2000). The high prevalence of depression and dementia in elder abuse or neglect. *Journal of the American Geriatrics Society, 48*(2), 205–208.

Feinberg, L. F. (2006). How far has family caregiving come? A 30-year perspective. *Aging Today, 27*(4), 3–4.

Figueroa, A. (2003, Summer). Speaking of the unspeakable. *AARP Segunda Juventud.* Retrieved January 13, 2006, from http://www.aarpsegundajuventud.org/english/issues/2003-july/elder_abuse.htm

Fisher, B. S., & Regan, S. L. (2006). The extent and frequency of abuse in the lives of older women and their relationship with health outcomes. *The Gerontologist, 46*, 200–209.

Folstein, M. F., Folstein, S. E., & McHugh, P. R. (1975). Mini-mental state. *Journal of Psychiatric Research, 12*(3), 189–198.

Fox-Grage, W., Coleman, B., & Folkemer, D. (2004). *The states' response to the Olmstead decision: A 2003 update.* Retrieved November 20, 2006, from http://www.ncsl.org/programs/health/forum/olmstead/2003/olms2003 report.htm

Fulmer, T., Firpo, A., Guadagno, L., Easter, T. M., Kahan, F., & Paris, B. (2003). Themes from a grounded theory analysis of elder neglect assessment by experts. *Gerontologist, 43*(5), 745–752.

Fulmer, T., Guadagno, L., Dyer, C. B., & Connolly, M. T. (2004). Progress in elder abuse screening and assessment instruments. *Journal of the American Geriatrics Society, 52*(2), 297–304.

Gallagher-Thompson, D. (1994). Direct services and interventions for caregivers: A review of extant programs and a look to the future. In M. A. Cantor (Ed.) *Family caregiving: Agenda for the future.* San Francisco: American Society on Aging.

Gallo, J. J. (2006). *Handbook of geriatric assessment* (4th ed.). Sudbury, MA: Jones and Bartlett Publishers.

Ganley, A. L. (1981). *Court-mandated counseling for men who batter: A three-day workshop for health professionals, participant's manual.* Washington D.C.: Center for Women Policy Studies.

Gelles, R. J., & Loseke, D. R. (Eds.). (1993). *Current controversies on family violence.* Newbury Park, CA: Sage Publications.

Giacomazzi, A., & Smithey, M. (2001). Community policing and family violence against women: Lessons learned from a multiagency collaborative. *Police Quarterly, 4*(1), 99–122.

Golden, G. S. (2004). Forensic odontology and elder abuse—a case study. *Journal of the California Dental Association, 32*(4), 336–340.

Grafstrom, M., Nordberg, A., & Winblad, B. (1992). Abuse is in the eye of the beholder. Report by family members about abuse of demented persons in home care. A total population-based study. *Scandinavian Journal of Social Medicine, 21*(4), 247–255.

Greenberg, J., et al. (1990). Dependent adult children & elder abuse. *Journal of Elder Abuse & Neglect, 2*(1/2), 73–86.

Griffin, L. W., & Williams, O. J. (1992). Abuse among African-American elderly. *Journal of Family Violence, 7*(1), 19–35.

Groh, A. (2003). *A healing approach to elder abuse and mistreatment: The restorative justice approaches to elder abuse project.* Retrieved August 29, 2007, from http://www.crnetwork.ca/about/include/ElderAbuseManual.pdf

Guion, L. A., Turner, J., & Wise, D. K. (2004). Design, implementation, and evaluation of an elder financial abuse program [Electronic version]. *Journal of Extension, 42*(3).

Hafemeister, T. L. (2003). Financial abuse of the elderly in domestic settings. In R. J. Bonnie & R. B. Wallace (Eds.), *Elder mistreatment: Abuse neglect and exploitation in an aging America* (pp. 382–445). Washington D.C.: National Academies Press.

Hamberger, L. K., & Potente, T. P. (1996). Counseling heterosexual women arrested for domestic violence: Implications for theory and practice. In C. M. Renzetti & L. K Hamberger, (Eds.), *Domestic partner abuse.* Springer Publishing Company.

Hamilton, G. P. (1989). Prevent elder abuse: Using a family systems approach. *Journal of Gerontological Nursing, 15*(3), 21–26.

Hankin, M. (1996). Making the perpetrator pay: Collecting damages for elder abuse, neglect and exploitation. *Aging, 367,* 66–70.

Hansberry, M. R., Chen, E., & Gorbien, M. J. (2005). Dementia and elder abuse. *Clinics in Geriatric Medicine, 21*(2), 315–332.

Harrison, P. M., & Karberg, J. C. (2003). *Prison and jail inmates at midyear 2002 (NCJ-198877).* Washington D.C.: Bureau of Justice Statistics, U.S. Department of Justice.

Hargrave, R. (2006). AGS position paper: Caregivers of African-American elderly with dementia: A review and analysis. *Annals of Long-Term Care, 14*(10), 36–40.

Hawes, C. (2003). Elder abuse in residential care settings: What is known and what information is needed? In R. J. Bonnie & R. B. Wallace (Eds.), *Elder mistreatment: Abuse neglect, and exploitation in an aging America* (pp. 446–500). Washington D.C.: National Academies Press.

Heath, J. M., Brown, M., Kobylarz, F. A., & Castaño, S. (2005). The prevalence of undiagnosed geriatric health conditions among adult protective service clients. *The Gerontologist, 45,* 820–823.

Heisler, C. J., & Quinn, M. J. (1995). A legal perspective. *Journal of Elder Abuse & Neglect, 7*(2/3), 131–156.

Heisler, C. J., & Stiegel, L. (2002). Enhancing the justice system's response to elder abuse: Discussions and recommendations of the "Improving Prosecution" working group of the National Policy Summit on Elder Abuse. *Journal of Elder Abuse & Neglect, 14*(4), 31–54.

Henningsen, E. J. (2000). Preventing financial abuse by agents under powers of attorney. *Wisconsin Lawyer 73*(9). Retrieved November 22, 2006, from http://www.wisbar.org/wislawmag/2000/09/henning.html

Hightower, J. (2002). *Violence and abuse in the lives of older women: Is it elder abuse or violence against women? Does it make any difference? Gender aspects of violence and abuse of older persons.* Background Paper for INSTRAW Electronic Discussion Forum, April 15–26, 2002.

Holland, G. B. (1985). *For Sasha, with love: An Alzheimer's crusade, the Anne Bashkiroff story.* New York: Red Dember Enterprises.

Homer, A. C., & Gilleard, C. (1990). Abuse of elderly people by their careers. *British Medical Journal, 301*(6765), 1359–1362.

Hounsell, C., & Riojas, A. M. (2006). Older women face tarnished "golden years" [Electronic version]. *Aging Today, 27*(2), 7, 9.

Hudson, M. F., & Carlson, J. R. (1999). Elder abuse: Its meaning to Caucasians, African Americans, and Native Americans. In T. Tatara (Ed.), *Understanding elder abuse in minority populations* (pp. 187–204). Philadelphia: Brunner/Mazel.

Hughes, M. (2000). *Remedying abuse by financial agents. Wisconsin Lawyer, 73 (9).* Retrieved November 22, 2006, from http://www.wisbar.org/wislawmag/2000/09/hughes.html

Humane Society of the United States. (n.d.). *Elder abuse and animal cruelty.* Retrieved December 8, 2006, from http://www.hsus.org/hsus_field/first_strike_the_connection_between_animal_cruelty_and_human_violence/elder_abuse_and_animal_cruelty/

Ingram, E. (2003). Expert panel recommendations on elder mistreatment using a public health framework. *Journal of Elder Abuse & Neglect, 15*(2), 45–65.

Jacoby L. L., Bishara, A. J., Hessels, S., & Toth, J. P. (2005). Aging, subjective experience, and cognitive control: Dramatic false remembering by older adults. *Journal of Experimental Psychology, 134*(2), 131–148.

Jasinski, J. L., & Dietz, T. (2003). Domestic violence and stalking among older adults: An assessment of risk markers. *Journal of Elder Abuse & Neglect, 15*(1), 3–18.

Javelin Strategy and Research. (2005). *The 2005 identity fraud survey report.* Retrieved July 18, 2005, from http://www.javelinstrategy.com/reports/documents/2005_Javeln_Strategy_Research_Identity_Fraud_Survey_Complimentary_Report.pdf

Jeary, K. (2004). Sexual abuse of elderly people: Would we rather not know the details? *Journal of Adult Protection, 6*(2), 21–30.

Jewkes, R (2002). Intimate partner violence: Causes and prevention. *Lancet, 359*(9315), 1423–1425.

Jogerst, G. J., Daly, J. M., Brinig, M. F., Dawson, J. D., Schmuch, G. A., & Ingram, J. G. (2003). Domestic elder abuse and the law. *American Journal of Public Health, 93*(12), 2131–2136.

Jogerst, G., Daly, J., & Ingram, J. (2001). National elder abuse questionnaire: Summary of adult protective service investigator responses. *Journal of Elder Abuse & Neglect, 13*(4), 59–71.

Johnson, T. (1986). Critical issues in the definition of elder mistreatment. In K. Pillemer & R. Wolf (Eds.), *Elder abuse: Conflict in the family* (pp. 167–196). Dover, MA: Auburn.

Jones, B.J. (2000). Role of Indian tribal courts in the justice system. Part of the series Native American Topic-specific monograph project. University of Oklahoma Health Science Center. Retrieved August 25, 2007, from the World Wide Web: www.icctc.org/Tribal Courts-final.pdf

Kane, R. L., Ouslander, J. G., & Abrass, I. B. (1994). *Essentials of clinical geriatrics* (3rd ed.). New York: McGraw-Hill.

Kapp, M. B. (1995). Elder mistreatment: Legal interventions and policy uncertainties. *Behavioral Sciences and the Law, 13*(3), 365–380.

Karp, N., & Wood, E. (2003). *Incapacitated and alone: Health care decision-making for the unbefriended elderly.* Washington D.C.: American Bar Association.

Karp, N., & Wood, E. (2006). *Guardianship monitoring: A national survey of court practices.* Washington D.C.: AARP.

Kaul, A., & Duffy, S. (1991). Gerontophilia—a case report. *Medicine, Science and the Law, 31*(2), 110–114.

Kelly, S., & Blythe, B. J. (2000). Family preservation: A potential not yet realized. *Child Welfare, 79,* 29–42.

Kleinschmidt, K. C. (1997). Elder abuse: A review. *Annals of Internal Medicine, 30*(4), 463–472.

Koenig, T. L., Rinfrette, E. S., & Lutz, W. A. (2006). Female caregivers' reflections on ethical decision-making: The intersection between domestic violence and elder abuse. *Clinical Social Work Journal, 34*(3), 361–372.

Koin, D. (2003). A forensic medical examination form for improved documentation and prosecution of elder abuse. *Journal of Elder Abuse & Neglect, 15*(3/4), 109–119.

Kosberg, J. (1998). Abuse of elderly men. *Journal of Elder Abuse & Neglect, 9*(3), 69–88.

Koss, M. P., Bachar, K. J., & Hopkins, C. Q. (2003). Restorative justice for sexual violence: Repairing victims, building community, and holding offenders accountable. *Annals of the New York Academy of Sciences, 989,* 384–396.

Kozak, J. F. (1994). Difficulties in addressing abuse and neglect in elderly patients. *Canadian Medical Association Journal, 151*(10), 1401–1403.

Kristof, K. M. (October 8, 2006). Law students to the rescue. *Los Angeles Times.*

Kurki, L. (1999). *Incorporating restorative and community justice into American sentencing and corrections. Research in brief.* Retrieved November 17, 2006, from http://www.ncjrs.gov/txtfiles1/nij/175723.txt

Kurki, L. (2003). Evaluating restorative justice practice. In A. von Hirsch, J. Roberts, & A. Bottoms (Eds.), *Restorative justice and criminal justice: Competing or reconcilable paradigms?* (pp. 293–314). Oxford: Hart Publishing.

Lachs, M. S., Berkman, L., Fulmer, T., & Horwitz, R. I. (1994). A prospective community-based pilot study of risk factors for the investigation of elder mistreatment. *Journal of the American Geriatrics Society, 42*(2), 169–173.

Lachs, M. S., & Pillemer, K. (1995). Abuse and neglect of elderly persons. *New England Journal of Medicine, 332*(7), 437–443.

Lachs, M. S., & Pillemer, K. (2004). Elder abuse. *Lancet, 364*(9441), 1263–1272.

Lachs, M. S., Williams, C., O'Brien, S., Hurst, L., & Horwitz, R. (1996). Older adults. An 11-year longitudinal study of adult protective service use. *Archives of Internal Medicine, 156*(4), 449–453.

Lauder, W. (1999). A survey of self-neglect in patients living in the community. *Journal of Clinical Nursing, 8*(1), 95–102.

Layton, M. J. (July 24, 2001). 400 home health aides fail state crime check: But most have passed back-ground review. *The Record*, pp. A-1, A-9.

Letellier, R. (1994). Gay and bisexual male domestic violence victimization: Challenges to feminist theory and responses to violence. *Violence and Victims, 9*(2), 95–106.

Lindbloom, E., J., Brandt, C., Hawes, C., Phillips, D., Zimmerman, J., Robinson, B., et al. (April 2005). *The role of forensic science in identification of mistreatment deaths in long-term care facilities.* Final report submitted to the National Institute of Justice (NCJ 209334). Available from http://www.ncjrs.gov/pdffiles1/nij/grants/209334.pdf

Lingler, J. (2003). Ethical issues in distinguishing sexual activity from sexual maltreatment among women with dementia. *Journal of Elder Abuse & Neglect, 15*(2), 85–102.

Macolini, R. M. (1995). Elder abuse policy: Considerations in research and legislation. *Behavioral Sciences & the Law, 13*(3), 349–363.

Malks, B., Buckmaster, J., & Cunningham, L. (2003). Combating elder financial abuse: A multi-disciplinary approach to a growth problem. *Journal of Elder Abuse & Neglect, 15*(3/4), 55–70.

Malley-Morrison, K. (Ed.). (2004). *International perspectives on family violence and abuse: A cognitive ecological approach.* Mahwah, NJ: Lawrence Erlbaum Associates.

Marshall, T. F. (1999). Restorative justice: An overview. Retrieved June 23, 2007, from http://www.homeoffice.gov.uk/rds/pdfs/occ-resjus.pdf

Maruna, S., & Copes, H. (2005). What have we learned in five decades of neutralization research? *Crime and Justice: A Review of Research, 32*, 221–320.

Matthias, R. E., & Benjamin, A. E. (2003). Abuse and neglect of clients in agency-based and consumer-directed home care. *Health & Social Work, 28*(3), 174–184.

Maxwell, C., Garner, J., & Fagan, J. (2002). The preventive effects of arrest on intimate partner violence: Research, policy and theory. *Criminology & Public Policy, 2*(1), 51–80.

Maxwell, E. K., & Maxwell, R. J. (1992). Insults to the body civil: Mistreatment of elderly in two Plains Indian tribes. *Journal of Cross-Cultural Gerontology, 7*(1), 3–23.

McDaniel, S. H., Lusterman, D.-D., & Philpot, C. L. (2001). *Casebook for integrating family therapy: An ecosystemic approach* (1st ed.). Washington D.C.: American Psychological Association.

McIntosh, S. (2002). *The links between animal abuse and family violence, as reported by women entering shelters in Calgary communities.* Calgary, AB: Author.

McNamee, C. C., & Murphy, M. B. (2006, November). Elder abuse in the United States. *NIJ Journal, 225.* Retrieved December 5, 2006, from http://www.ojp.usdoj.gov/nij/journals/255/elder_abuse.html

Meddaugh, D. I. (1993). Covert elder abuse in the nursing home. *Journal of Elder Abuse & Neglect, 5*(3), 21–37.

Meeks-Sjostrom, D. (2004). A comparison of three measures of elder abuse. *Journal of Nursing Scholarship, 36*(3), 247–250.

Menio, D. A. (1996). Advocating for the rights of vulnerable nursing home residents: Creative strategies. *Journal of Elder Abuse & Neglect, 8*(3), 59–72.

Miller, S. L. (1994). Expanding the boundaries: Toward a more inclusive and integrated study of intimate violence. *Violence and Victims, 9*(2), 183–194.

Miller, L. S., Clark, M., & Clark, W. F. (1998). The comparative evaluation of California's Multipurpose Senior Services Project. *Home Health Care Services Quarterly, 6*(3), 49–79.

Millet, K. (1971). *Sexual politics.* New York: Avon.

Mixson, P. M. (1995). An adult protective services perspective. *Journal of Elder Abuse & Neglect, 7*(2/3), 69–87.

Mixson, P. (2005). Canary in a coal mine? Part II. *Victimization of the Elderly and Disabled, 8*(3), 35.

Mixson, P. (2005). Tipping the balance in favor of protection. *Victimization of the Elderly and Disabled, 8*(4), 49–64.

Montgomery, R. J., & Kosloski, K. (2000). Family caregiving: Change, continuity, and diversity. In M. P. Lawton & R. Rubinstein (Eds.), *Interventions in dementia care: Toward improving quality of life* (pp. 143–172). New York: Springer.

Montoya, V. (1997). Understanding and combating elder abuse in Hispanic communities. *Journal of Elder Abuse & Neglect, 9*(2), 5–17.

Moody, H. R. (1988). From informed consent to negotiated consent. *The Gerontologist, 28,* 64–70.

Moon, A., Tomita, S., Talamantes, M. S., Brown, A., Sanchez, Y., Benton, D., et al. (1998). *Attitudes toward elder mistreatment and reporting: A multicultural study.* Washington D.C.: National Center on Elder Abuse.

Moon, A., & Williams, O. (1993). Perceptions of elder abuse and help-seeking patterns among African-American, Caucasian American, and Korean-American elderly women. *Gerontologist, 33*(3), 386–395.

Morgan, S. P., & Scott, J. M. (2003). *Prosecution of elder abuse, neglect, & exploitation: Criminal liability, due process and hearsay.* Alexandria, VA: American Prosecutors Research Institute.

Moskowitz, S. (1998). New remedies for elder abuse and neglect. *Probate and Property, 12,* 52–56.

Moskowitz, S. (2001). Filial responsibility statutes: Legal and policy considerations. *Journal of Law and Policy, 9*(3), 709–736.

Moskowitz, S. (2003). Golden age in the golden state: Contemporary legal developments in elder abuse and neglect. *Loyola Law Review, 36*(2), 589–666.

Mosqueda, L., Burnight, K., & Liao, S. (2005). The life cycle of bruises in older adults. *Journal of the American Geriatrics Society, 53*, 1339–1343.

Mosqueda, L., Burnight, K., Liao, S., & Kemp, B. (2004). Advancing the field of elder mistreatment: A new model for integration of social and medical services. *Gerontologist, 44*(5), 703–708.

Murray, M., & O'Ran, S. (2002). *Restitution*. Retrieved June 19, 2007, from http://www.ojp.usdoj.gov/ovc/assist/nvaa2002/chapter5_1.html

Myers, J. E. B. (2005). *Myers on evidence in child, domestic, and elder abuse*: New York. Aspen Publishers, Inc.

Myers, R., & Jacobo, J. (2005). Sex offenders in nursing homes. *Victimization of the Elderly and Disabled, 7*(6), 85–86.

Naimark, D. (2001). Financial exploitation of the elderly: The evaluation of mental capacity and undue influence. *American Journal of Forensic Psychiatry, 22*(3), 5–19.

National Adult Protective Services Association. *Code of ethics*. Retrieved December 6, 2006, from http://www.apsnetwork.org/About/ethics.htm

National Association of State Units on Aging. (2006). *Strategy brief: Ombudsman program advocacy in guardianship. Report on national dialogue forum #4*. Retrieved April 17, 2007, from www.nasua.org/pdf/Strat.%20Brief%20 Advocacy%20in%20Guardianship.pdf

National Center for Victims of Crime. (1999). *Elder abuse and the law*. Retrieved May 21, 2007, from http://www.ncvc.org/ncvc/main.aspx?dbName=Document Viewer&DocumentAction=ViewProperties&DocumentID=32465&UrlTo Return=http%3a%2f%2fwww.ncvc.org%2fncvc%2fmain.aspx%

National Center on Elder Abuse. (1998). *The National Elder Abuse Incidence Study, Final Report*. Washington D.C.: The National Center on Elder Abuse.

National Center on Elder Abuse. (2003). Law enforcement, justice, and adult protective services team up in Pennsylvania. *NCEA Newsletter, 5*(7).

National Institute on Aging. (Aug 29, 2006). *Review of minority aging research at the NIA*. Retrieved January 16, 2007, from http://www.nia.nih.gov/ AboutNIA/MinorityAgingResearch.htm

National Institute of Mental Health. (2001). *Post-traumatic stress disorder*. Retrieved April 1, 2007, from http://www.nimh.nih.gov/publicat/reliving.cfm

National Research Council. (2003). *Elder mistreatment: Abuse, neglect, and exploitation in an aging America*. Washington D.C.: National Academies Press.

Neale, A. V., Hwalek, M. A., Scott, R. O., Sengstock, M. C., & Stahl, C. (1991). Validation of the Hwalek-Sengstock elder abuse screening test. *Journal of Applied Gerontology, 10*(4), 406–418.

Nelson, H., Nygren, P., McInerney, Y., & Klein, J. (2004). Screening women and elderly adults for family and intimate partner violence: A Review of the evidence for the U.S. Preventive Services Task Force. *Annals of Internal Medicine, 140*(5), 387–404.

Nerenberg, L. (1995). Domestic violence advocate speaks out on elder abuse. *nexus: A publication for Affiliates of the National Committee for the Prevention of Elder Abuse, 1*(3), 7.

Nerenberg, L. (1996). Hornswoggled? An interview with Margaret Singer on undue influence. *nexus: A publication for affiliates of the National Committee for the Prevention of Elder Abuse,* 2(1), 4–6.

Nerenberg, L. (1999). *Forgotten victims of elder financial crime and abuse: A report and recommendations.* Retrieved December 14, 2006, from http://www.elderabusecenter.org/pdf/publication/fvefca.pdf

Nerenberg, L. (1999). Moving beyond violence: Treating older batterers. *nexus: A publication for Affiliates of the National Committee for the Prevention of Elder Abuse,* 5(1), 1, 4–6.

Nerenberg, L. (2000). Elder abuse & substance abuse: Making the connection [Interview with Charmaine Spencer and Jeff Smith]. *nexus: A Publication for NCPEA Affiliates,* 6(1), 1, 4–5, 7.

Nerenberg, L. (2000). *Helping Hands: The role of adult protective services in preventing elder abuse and neglect.* Washington, DC: National Center on Elder Abuse.

Nerenberg, L. (2001). Rich heritage: No shield against abuse. Marta Sotomayor, Ph.D. talks about elder abuse in the Latino community. *nexus: A publication for Affiliates of the National Committee for the Prevention of Elder Abuse,* 7(1), 1, 3, 4, 7.

Nerenberg, L. (2002a). Preventing elder abuse by in-home helpers. Washington D.C.: National Center on Elder Abuse.

Nerenberg, L. (2002b). The national policy summit issue briefs. *Journal of Elder Abuse & Neglect,* 14(4), 71–104.

Nerenberg, L. (2002c). Caregiver stress and elder abuse: Preventing elder abuse by family caregivers. Retrieved June 22, 2007, from http://www.elderabusecenter.org/pdf/family/caregiver.pdf [PDF:734kb]

Nerenberg, L. (2003). *Daily money management programs; A protection against elder abuse.* San Francisco: Institute on Aging.

Nerenberg, L. (2004). *Multidisciplinary elder abuse prevention teams: A new generation.* Washington D.C.: National Center on Elder Abuse.

Nerenberg, L., Baldridge, D., & Benson, B. (2003). *Preventing and responding to abuse of elders in Indian country.* Retrieved December 20, 2006, from http://www.elderabusecenter.org/pdf/whatnew/abuseindian040707.pdf

Nerenberg, L., & Njeri, M. (1993). WE ARE FAMILY: Outreach to African-American seniors. *Journal of Elder Abuse & Neglect,* 5(4), 5–19.

Neysmith, S. (1995). Power in relationships of trust: A feminist analysis of elder abuse. In M. J. MacLean (Ed.) *Abuse and neglect of older Canadians: Strategies for change.* Toronto: Thompson Educational Publishers, Inc.

Older Women's Network (Ontario) Inc. *Shelter needs of abused older women: Key findings and recommendations.* Retrieved November 20, 2006, from http://www.olderwomensnetwork.org/shelterneeds.htm

Olinger, P. (1991). The outlook for federal legislation. *Journal of Elder Abuse & Neglect,* 3(1), 43–52.

Olmstead v. L. C. (98–536) 527 U.S. 581 (1999).

Otto, J. M. (2000). The role of adult protective services in addressing abuse. *Generations,* 24(2), 33–38.

Otto, J., & Bell, J. (2003). *Problems facing state adult protective services programs and the resources needed to resolve them.* National Association of Adult Protective Services Administrators.

Patterson, M., & Malley-Morrison, K. (2006). A cognitive-ecological approach to elder abuse in five cultures: Human rights and education. *Educational Gerontology, 32,* 73–82.

Paveza, G. (2002). The elder justice bill's impact on research: Likely fact or fiction. *Journal of Elder Abuse & Neglect, 14*(2/3), 199–207.

Paveza, G. J., Cohen, D., Eisdorfer, C., Freels, S., Semla, T., Ashford, J. W., et al. (1992). Severe family violence and Alzheimer's disease: Prevalence and risk factors. *Gerontologist, 32*(4), 493–497.

Payne, B. (2003). Preventing elder abuse requires an integrated approach. *Quest, 6*(2).

People v. Heitzman, 9 Cal. 4th 189, 37 Cal. Rptr. 2d 236, 886 P. 2d 1229 (1994).

Perfect Cause, A. (2005). *Predators in America's nursing homes: 2005 report.* Retrieved January 7, 2007, from http://www.aperfectcause.com/PDF_APC/ APerfectCause-PredatorsinAmericasNursingHomes-2005Report.pdf

Pillemer, K., & Finkelhor, D. (1988). The prevalence of elder abuse: A random sample survey. *Gerontologist, 28*(1), 51–57.

Pillemer, K. A., & Moore, D. W. (1989). Abuse of patients in nursing homes: Findings from a survey of staff. *Gerontologist, 29*(3), 314–320.

Pillemer, K. A., & Suitor, J. J. (1992). Violence and violent feelings: What causes them among family caregivers? *Journal of Gerontology, 47*(4), S165–S172.

Pinquart, M., & Sörensen, S. (2005). Ethnic differences in stressors, resources, and psychological outcomes of family caregiving: A meta-analysis. *The Gerontologist, 45,* 90–106.

Podnieks, E. (1992). National survey on abuse of the elderly in Canada. *Journal of Elder Abuse & Neglect, 4*(1/2), 5–58.

Podnieks, E. (1999). Support groups: A chance at human connection for abused older adults. In J. Pritchard (Ed.), *Elder abuse work: Best practice in Britain and Canada* (pp. 457–483). London: Jessica Kinksley Publishers.

Podnieks, E., & Baillie, E. (1995). Education as the key to the prevention of elder abuse and neglect. In M. J. MacLean (Ed.), *Abuse & Neglect of Older Canadians: Strategies for Change* (pp. 81–93). Toronto, ON: Thompson Educational Publishing, Inc.

Podnieks, E., & Pillemer, K. (1990). *National survey on abuse of the elderly in Canada.* Toronto, ON: Ryerson Polytechnic University.

Podnieks, E., & Wilson, S. (2003). Elder abuse awareness in faith communities: Findings from a Canadian pilot study. *Journal of Elder Abuse & Neglect, 15*(3/4), 121–135.

Presser, L., & Gaarder, E. (2000). Can restorative justice reduce battering? Some preliminary considerations. *Social Justice, 27*(1), 175–195.

Quayhagen, M., Quayhagen, M., Patterson, T., Irwin, M., Hauger, R., & Grant, I. (1997). Coping with dementia: Family caregiver burnout and abuse. *Journal of Mental Health and Aging, 3*(3), 357–364.

Quinn, M. J. (2005). *Guardianships of adults: Achieving justice, autonomy, and safety*. New York: Springer.

Quinn, M. J., & Nerenberg, L. (2005). *Improving access to the San Francisco Superior Court (Probate and Unified Family Courts) for elders: Final report*. San Francisco: San Francisco Superior Court.

Quinn, M. J., & Tomita, S. K. (1997). *Elder abuse and neglect: Causes, diagnosis, and intervention strategies* (2 ed.). New York: Springer.

Rabiner, D. J., O'Keeffe, J., & Brown, D. (2006). Financial exploitation of older persons: Challenges and opportunities to identify, prevent, and address it in the United States. *Journal of Aging & Social Policy, 18*(2).

Ramsey-Klawsnik, H. (2004). Elder sexual abuse perpetrated by residents in care settings. *Victimization of the Elderly and Disabled, 6*(6), 81, 93–95.

Raye, B. E., & Roberts, A. W. (2004). A vision of justice. *ACResolution: The Quarterly Magazine of the Association for Conflict Resolution, 3*(4), 9–13.

Raymond, J. (2002). Building a statewide network of services for older abused women. *nexus: A publication for Affiliates of the National Committee for the Prevention of Elder Abuse, 8*(1 & 2), 11–12.

Reay, A., & Browne, K. (2002). The effectiveness of psychological interventions with individuals who physically abuse or neglect their elderly dependents. *Journal of Interpersonal Violence, 17*(4), 416–431.

Reis, M., & Nahmiash, D. (1998). Validation of the indicators of abuse (IOA) screen. *Gerontologist, 38*(4), 471–480.

Ridgway, M. L. (n.d.). *Civil, criminal and administration remedies in cases of abuse, neglect and financial exploitation of the elderly*. Retrieved June 19, 2007, from http://senioranswers.org/Pages/elderabuse.htm

Rittman, M., Kuzmeskus, L. B., & Flum, M. A. (1999). A synthesis of current knowledge on minority elder abuse. In T. Tatara (Ed.), *Understanding elder abuse in minority populations* (pp. 221–238). Philadelphia: Taylor & Francis.

Roby, J. L., & Sullivan, R. (2001). Adult protection service laws: A comparison of state statutes from definition to case closure. *Journal of Elder Abuse & Neglect, 12*(3/4), 17–51.

Rothman, M. B., & Dunlop, B. D. (2006). Elders and the courts: Judicial policy for an aging America. *Journal of Aging & Social Policy, 18*(2).

Rosenblatt, D. E., Cho, K. H., & Durance, P. W. (1996). Reporting mistreatment of older adults: The role of physicians. *Journal of the American Geriatrics Society, 44*(1), 65–70.

Royall, D. R., Mahurin, R. K., & Gray, K. F. (1992). Bedside assessment of executive cognitive impairment: The executive interview. *Journal of the American Geriatrics Society, 40*(12), 1221–1226.

Sacks, D. (1994). Elderly financial management project: Year one report. New York: Jacob Reingold Institute, Brookdale Center on Aging of Hunter College.

Schechter, S., & Ganley, A. L. (1995). *Domestic violence: A curriculum for family preservation practitioners*. San Francisco: Family Violence Prevention Fund.

Schiamberg, L. B., & Gans, D. (1999). Elder abuse by adult children: An applied ecological framework for understanding contextual risk factors and the intergenerational character of the quality of life. *International Journal of Aging and Human Development, 50,* 329–359.

Scogin, F., Beall C., Bynum, J., Stephens, G., Grote, N., Baumhover, L. A., et al. (1989). Training for abusive caregivers: An unconventional approach to an intervention dilemma. *Journal of Elder Abuse & Neglect, 1*(4), 73–85.

Seaver, C. (1996). Muted lives: Older battered women. *Journal of Elder Abuse & Neglect, 8*(2), 3–21.

Sherman, L. W., & Berk, R. A. (1984). The specific deterrent effects of arrest for domestic assault. *American Sociological Review, 49.*

Sherman, L. W., Schmidt, J. D., Rogan, D. P., Gartin, P. R., Cohn, E. G., Collins, D. J., et al. (1991). From initial deterrence to longterm escalation: Short-custody arrest for poverty ghetto domestic violence. *Criminology, 29*(4), 821–850.

Shipler, L. K., Anand, R., & Hadi, N. (1998). *Cultural considerations in assisting victims of crime: report on needs and promising practices.* Washington D.C.: National MultiCultural Institute.

Simpson, A. R. (2005). Cultural issues and elder mistreatment. *Clinics in Geriatric Medicine, 21*(2), 355–364.

Sonkin, D. J., & Durphy, M. (1982). *Learning to live without violence.* San Francisco: Volcano Press.

Sonkin, D. J., Martin D., & Walker, L. (1985).The male batterer: A treatment approach. New York: Springer.

Spencer, C. (1995). New directions for research on interventions with abused older adults. In M. J. MacLean (Ed.), *Abuse & neglect of older Canadians: Strategies for change* (pp. 143–155). Toronto, ON: Thompson Educational Publishing, Inc.

Squillace, M. R., & Firman, J. (2004). *The myths and realities of consumer-directed services for older persons.* Retrieved December 6, 2006, from http://www.consumerdirection.org/reso_mandr.php

Stanford, E. P. (1998). Diversity in an aging society: Abuse the wild card. In The Archstone Foundation (Ed.), *Understanding and combating elder abuse in minority communities* (pp. 19–24). Long Beach, CA: Archstone Foundation.

Stein, E. (2001). *Quantifying the economic cost of predatory lending.* Retrieved May 18, 2007, from http://www.responsiblelending.org/pdfs/Quant10-01.pdf

Stein, R. (July 28, 2003). Legal system struggles with dementia patients. *The Washington Post,* p A01.

Stiegel, L. (1995). *Recommended guidelines for state courts handling cases involving elder abuse.* Washington, D.C.: American Bar Association.

Stiegel, L. (2005). *Elder abuse fatality review teams: A replication manual.* Washington D.C.: American Bar Association.

Strang, H., & Braithwaite, J. (Eds.). (2002). *Restorative justice and family violence.* Melbourne: Cambridge University Press.

Sullivan, C. M., & Bybee, D. I. (1999). Reducing violence using community based advocacy for women with abusive partners. *Journal of Consulting and Clinical Psychology, 67*(1), 43–53.

Sykes, G., & Matza, D. (1957). Techniques of neutralization: A theory of delinquency. *American Sociological Review, 22*(6), 664–670.

Tatara, T. (1995). *An analysis of state laws addressing elder abuse, neglect, and exploitation.* Washington D.C.: National Center for Elder Abuse.

Tatara, T. (1999). *Understanding elder abuse in minority populations.* Philadelphia: Brunner/Mazel.

Tauriac, J., & Scruggs, N. (2006). Elder abuse among African Americans. *Educational Gerontology, 32*(1), 37–48.

Teaster, P. B., Dugar, T. A., Mendiondo, M. S., Abner, E. L., & Cecil, K. A. (2006). *The 2004 survey of state adult protective services: Abuse of adults 60 years of age and older.* Retrieved July 20, 2006, from http://www.elder abusecenter.org/pdf/2-14-06%20FINAL%2060+REPORT.pdf

Teaster, P. B., Lawrence, S. A., & Cecil, K. A. (2007). Elder abuse and neglect. *Aging Health, 3*(2), 115–128.

Teaster, P. B., & Nerenberg, L. (2003). *A national look at elder abuse multidisciplinary teams.* Washington D.C.: National Committee for the Prevention of Elder Abuse.

Teaster, P. B., & Roberto, K. A. (2004). Sexual abuse of older adults: APS cases and outcomes. *Gerontologist, 44*(6), 788–796.

Teaster, P. B., Wood, E. F., Karp, N., Lawrence, S. A., Schmidt, W. C., & Mendiondo, M. S. (2005). *Wards of the state: A national study of public guardianship.* Retrieved April 17, 2007, from http://www.mc.uky.edu/ gerontology/Research%20Reports/Wards%20of%20State%20Public% 20Guardianship%20final%20copy.pdf

Tomita, S. K. (1990). The denial of elder mistreatment by victims and abusers: The application of neutralization theory. *Violence & Victims, 5*(3), 171–184.

Tomita, S. (1994). The consideration of cultural factors in the research of elder mistreatment with an in-depth look at the Japanese. *Journal of Cross-Cultural Gerontology, 9*, 39–52.

Tomita, S. (2006). Mistreated and neglected elders. In B. Berkman (Ed.), *Handbook of social work in health and aging* (pp. 219–230). New York: Oxford.

Torres-Gil, F. (1998). Keynote speech: The social context of aging. In The Archstone Foundation (Ed.), *Understanding and combating elder abuse in minority communities* (pp. 7–8). Long Beach, CA: The Archstone Foundation.

Tyra, P. (1996). Helping elderly women survive rape using a crisis framework. *Journal of Psychosocial Nursing & Mental Health Services, 34*(12), 20–25.

United Nations Economic and Social Council. (February 25–March 1, 2002). *Abuse of older persons: Recognizing and responding to abuse of older persons in a global context.* New York, NY: Document of the Commission for Social Development.

U.S. Department of Health and Human Services, Administration on Aging. (2006). *Profile of Older Americans: 2006.* Retrieved August 28, 2007, from http://www.aoa.gov/prof/statistics/profile/2006/2006profile.pdf

U.S. Department of Health and Human Services, Office of Disability, Aging and Long-Term Care Policy. (2006). *Ensuring a qualified long-term care workforce: From pre-employment screens to on-the-job monitoring.* Retrieved February 14, 2007, from http://aspe.hhs.gov/daltcp/reports/2006/LTCW qual.htm

U.S. Department of Justice. (1998). *Guidelines for the screening of persons work-ing with children, the elderly, and individuals with disabilities in need of support* (NCJ 167248). Retrieved February 7, 2007, from http://www.ncjrs. gov/pdffiles/167248.pdf

U.S. Department of Justice, Office for Victims of Crime. (1998). *New directions from the field: Victims' rights and services for the 21st century.* Washington D.C.: U.S. Department of Justice, Office of Justice Programs, Office for Victims of Crime.

U.S. Department of Justice, Office for Victims of Crime. (1999). *Promising victim-related practices in probation and parole.* Retrieved May 21, 2007, from http://www.ojp.usdoj.gov/ovc/publications/infores/probparole/welcome.html

U.S. Department of Justice, Office for Victims of Crime (2002a). *Making res-titution work.* Legal Series no. 5. Retrieved December 28, 2005, from www.ojp.usdoj.gov/ovc/publications/bulletins/legalseries/bulletin5/ ncj189193.pdf

U.S. Department of Justice, Office for Victims of Crime. (2002b). *Victimization of the elderly. Chapter 14 of the National Victim Assistance Academy instruc-tors manual.* Retrieved March 8, 2007, from www.ojp.usdoj.gov/ovc/assist/ nvaa2002/chapter14.html

U.S. Government Accountability Office. (1996). *Long term care: Some states apply criminal background checks to home care workers.* Retrieved June 18, 2007, from http://frwebgate.access.gpo.gov/cgi-bin/getdoc.cgi?dbname= gao&docid=f:pe96005.txt

U.S. Government Accountability Office. (1999). *Nursing homes: Additional steps needed to strengthen enforcement of federal quality standards.* Retrieved June 19, 2007, from http://www.gao.gov/archive/1999/he99046.pdf

U.S. Government Accountability Office. (2002). *Nursing homes: More can be done to protect residents from abuse.* Washington D.C.: GAO-02-312. Retrieved April 19, 2007, from the World Wide Web: http://www.gao.gov/ new.items/d02312.pdf

U.S. Government Accountability Office. (2004). *Guardianships: Collaboration needed to protect incapacitated elderly people.* GAO-04-655. Retrieved June 22, 2007, from http://www.gao.gov/new.items/d04655.pdf

U.S. Government Accountability Office. (2005). *Criminal debt: Court ordered restitution amounts far exceed likely collections for the crime victims in selected financial fraud cases.* Retrieved June 18, 2006, from www.gao.gov/ cgi-bin/getrpt?GAO-05-80

U.S. Government Accountability Office. (2006). *Long-term care facilities: Infor-mation on residents who are registered sex offenders or paroled for other crimes.* Retrieved May 22, 2007, from http://www.gao.gov/highlights/ d06326high.pdf

U.S. House of Representatives, Subcommittee on Domestic and International Scientific Planning, Analysis, and Cooperation. (1978). Hearings of the Committee on Science and Technology, February 15. Washington D.C.: Government Printing Office.

U.S. House of Representatives, Subcommittee on Financial Institutions and Consumer Credit, and Subcommittee on Housing and Community Opportunity

Committee on Financial Services (June 23, 2004). Promoting home ownership by ensuring liquidity in the subprime mortgage market. Retrieved August 29, 2007, from http://a257.g.akamaitech.net/7/257/2422/06oct20041230/www.access.gpo.gov/congress/house/pdf/108hrg/95652.pdf

Vinton, L. (1998). A nationwide survey of domestic violence shelters' programming for older women. *Violence against Women, 4*, 559–571.

Walker, D. (2005). Michigan Elder Abuse Task Force: A short description of activities. *The Michigan Advocate, 6*(2).

Walters, N., & Hermanson, S. (2001). *Subprime mortgage lending and older borrowers*, from http://www.aarp.org/research/credit-debt/mortgages/aresearch-import-182-DD57.html

Websdale, N. (2000). *Lethality assessment tools: A critical analysis.* Retrieved December 23, 2006, from http://www.vawnet.org/DomesticViolence/Research/VAWnetDocs/AR_lethality.pdf

WHO/INPEA. (2002). *Missing voices: Views of older persons on elder abuse.* Retrieved December 20, 2006, from http://www.who.int/ageing/projects/elder_abuse/missing_voices/en/index.html.

Wilber, K. (1995). The search for effective alternatives to conservatorship: Lessons from a daily money management diversion study. *Journal of Aging & Social Policy, 7*(1), 39–56.

Wilber, K., & Cedano, K. A. (2002). Southern California Presbyterian Homes Financial Services Program. Annual evaluation report. Jan 1, 2001 – December 31, 2001. Los Angeles: University of Southern California.

Wilber, K., & Reynolds, S. L. (1996). Introducing a framework for defining financial abuse of the elderly. *Journal of Elder Abuse & Neglect, 8*(2), 61–80.

Williams-Burgess, C., & Kimball, M. J. (1992). The neglected elder: A family systems approach. *Journal of Psychosocial Nursing & Mental Health Services, 30*(10), 21–25.

Wolf, R. (1997). Elder abuse and neglect: Causes and consequences. *Journal of Geriatric Psychiatry, 30*(1), 153–174.

Wolf, R. (1999a). *A research agenda on abuse of older persons and adults with disabilities.* Retrieved May 8, 2007, from http://www.elderabusecenter.org/default.cfm?p=researchagenda.cfm

Wolf, R. (1999b). *Elder Shelters: U.S., Canada, and Japan.* Washington D.C.: National Center on Elder Abuse.

Wolf, R. (2000). Risk assessment instruments (Electronic version). *National Center on Elder Abuse Newsletter, 3*(1).

Wolf, R. S., & Pillemer, K. A. (1989). *Helping Elderly Victims: The Reality of ElderAbuse.* New York: Columbia University Press.

Wolf, R. S. (2001). Support groups for older victims of domestic violence. *Journal of Women & Aging, 13*(4), 71–83.

Wolf, R. S. (2003). Elder abuse and neglect: History and concepts. In R. J. Bonnie & R. B. Wallace (Eds.), *Elder mistreatment: Abuse, neglect, and exploitation in an aging America.* Washington D.C.: National Academies Press.

Wood, E. (2006). *The availability and utility of interdisciplinary data on elder abuse: A white paper for the National Center on Elder Abuse.* Retrieved

February 20, 2007, from http://www.elderabusecenter.org/pdf/publication/ WhitePaper060404.pdf

Zarit, S. H., & Toseland, R. W. (1989). Current and future direction in family caregiving research. *Gerontologist, 29,* 481–483.

Index

Page number followed by an italicized *t* indicates a table.

Index

Index

Index

Index

Index

Index

Index